CBD vs Kratom: 2 Books in 1: Your Ultimate Guide to Understanding and Using CBD Oil and Kratom

Frank Coles

Welcome to this 2 book bundle containing two of my best selling books on CBD Oil and Kratom.

This book bundle was designed to provide you with the most in-depth and up to date information about CBD Oil and Kratom.

From supporting you in understanding what the supplements are and where they come from to discovering why they are used and what side effects you may face when using them, this bundle contains everything. It truly is the most comprehensive guide on the market to support you in understanding CBD Oil and Kratom and how they can positively benefit you or your loved ones who are considering using them.

So, let us get right ahead and find out more about the wonders of CBD Oil and Kratom.

Copyright 2018 by Frank Coles - All rights reserved.

The following book is reproduced below with the goal of providing information that is as accurate and reliable as possible. Regardless, purchasing this book can be seen as consent to the fact that both the publisher and the author of this book are in no way experts on the topics discussed within and that any recommendations or suggestions that are made herein are for entertainment purposes only. Professionals should be consulted as needed prior to undertaking any of the action endorsed herein.

This declaration is deemed fair and valid by both the American Bar Association and the Committee of Publishers Association and is legally binding throughout the United States.

Furthermore, the transmission, duplication or reproduction of any of the following work including specific information will be considered an illegal act irrespective of if it is done electronically or in print. This extends to creating a secondary or tertiary copy of the work or a recorded copy and is only allowed with an expressed written consent from the Publisher. All additional rights reserved.

The information in the following pages is broadly considered to be a truthful and accurate account of facts and as such any inattention, use or misuse of the information in question by the reader will render any resulting actions solely under their purview. There are no scenarios in which the publisher or the original author of this work can be in any fashion deemed liable for any hardship or damages that may befall them after undertaking information described herein.

Additionally, the information in the following pages is intended only for informational purposes and should thus be thought of as universal. As befitting its nature, it is presented without assurance regarding its prolonged validity or interim quality. Trademarks that are mentioned are done without written consent and can in no way be considered an endorsement from the trademark holder.

Table of Contents

CBD: 101 Things You Need To Know About CBD Oil 19

Introduction 20

Chapter 1: What is CBD Oil? 22

What is CBD Oil? 22

1st thing you need know… 22

2nd thing you need know… 22

3rd thing you need know… 23

4th thing you need know...23

5th thing you need know...24

Where Does it Come From? 24

6th thing you need know...24

7th thing you need know...24

8th thing you need know...25

9th thing you need know...25

10th thing you need know.......................................25

11th thing you need know.......................................26

12th thing you need know.......................................26

What is A Cannabinoid? 27

13th thing you need know.......................................27

14th thing you need know………………………………27

Chapter 2: Why Should I Use CBD Oil? …………28

Why is CBD Oil Good For You? ……………………28

15th thing you need know………………………………28

16th thing you need know………………………………29

17th thing you need know………………………………29

18th thing you need know………………………………29

19th thing you need know………………………………30

20th thing you need know………………………………31

21st thing you need know… …………………………31

22nd thing you need know… …………………………31

23rd thing you need know………………………………32

24th thing you need know………………………………32

25th thing you need know………………………………33

Is it Safe? …………………………………………………33

26th thing you need know………………………………33

27th thing you need know………………………………34

28th thing you need know………………………………35

29th thing you need know………………………………35

30th thing you need know………………………………36

31st thing you need know… …………………………36

Common Uses……………………………………………37

32nd thing you need know... 37

33rd thing you need know..............................37

34th thing you need know..............................38

35th thing you need know..............................38

36th thing you need know..............................39

37th thing you need know..............................40

38th thing you need know..............................40

39th thing you need know..............................41

40th thing you need know..............................41

41st thing you need know... 42

42nd thing you need know... 43

43rd thing you need know..............................43

44th thing you need know..............................44

45th thing you need know..............................44

46th thing you need know..............................45

47th thing you need know..............................46

48th thing you need know..............................46

49th thing you need know..............................47

50th thing you need know..............................47

51st thing you need know... 48

52nd thing you need know... 48

Chapter 3: How Do I Take CBD Oil? 50

Topically 50

53rd thing you need know.......................... 50

54th thing you need know.......................... 50

55th thing you need know.......................... 51

56th thing you need know.......................... 51

57th thing you need know.......................... 52

58th thing you need know.......................... 52

59th thing you need know.......................... 53

Ingested.. 53

60th thing you need know.......................... 53

61st thing you need know... 54

62nd thing you need know... 54

63rd thing you need know.......................... 55

64th thing you need know.......................... 56

65th thing you need know.......................... 56

Vaporized 56

66th thing you need know.......................... 57

67th thing you need know.......................... 57

68th thing you need know.......................... 57

69th thing you need know.......................... 58

70th thing you need know.......................... 58

71st thing you need know... 59

72nd thing you need know… 60

73rd thing you need know…..................................60

Chapter 4: Who Should Take CBD Oil? 62

General Facts 62

74th thing you need know…..................................62

75th thing you need know…..................................63

Children 63

76th thing you need know…..................................63

77th thing you need know…..................................64

78th thing you need know…..................................65

79th thing you need know…..................................65

80th thing you need know…..................................66

Adults 66

81st thing you need know… 66

82nd thing you need know… 67

Seniors 67

83rd thing you need know…..................................68

84th thing you need know…..................................68

85th thing you need know…..................................69

86th thing you need know…..................................69

87th thing you need know…..................................70

Chapter 5: Side Effects of CBD Oil 71

Medicinal Considerations 71

88th thing you need know……...........................71

89th thing you need know……...........................72

90th thing you need know……...........................72

91st thing you need know… 72

Symptomatic Side Effects................................73

92nd thing you need know… 73

93rd thing you need know……............................73

94th thing you need know……...........................74

95th thing you need know……...........................74

96th thing you need know……...........................75

97th thing you need know……...........................75

98th thing you need know……...........................76

99th thing you need know……...........................76

100th thing you need know…............................77

101st thing you need know… 77

Conclusion 78

Kratom: 101 Things You Need To Know About Kratom………………………………………………………………..80

Introduction 81

Chapter 1: Kratom Knowledge: A Botanical Background 84

1st thing you need to know…............................84

2nd thing you need to know… 85

3rd thing you need to know… 85

4th thing you need to know… 86

5th thing you need to know… 87

6th thing you need to know… 87

7th thing you need to know… 88

Chemical Characteristics & Core Compound Constituents 88

8th thing you need to know… 88

9th thing you need to know… 89

10th thing you need to know… 90

Inherent Interactions 91

11th thing you need to know… 91

12th thing you need to know… 91

13th thing you need to know… 91

Chapter 2: Specific Strains 93

14th thing you need to know… 93

Clarifications in Colour Classification 93

15th thing you need to know… 94

16th thing you need to know… 94

17th thing you need to know… 95

Watery Whites 95

18th thing you need to know… 95

Generous Greens 96

19th thing you need to know… 96

Regional Reds 97

20th thing you need to know… 97

Stimulating Strains..98

21st thing you need to know…...............................98

Sedating Strains..99

22nd thing you need to know… 99

Chapter 3: Prescriptive Preparations & Ideal Ingestions 101

Leaf of Life 101

23rd thing you need to know…..............................101

Power Powder 102

24th thing you need to know…..............................102

25th thing you need to know…..............................103

Tea Treat 108

26th thing you need to know…..............................108

Exhilarating Extract...110

27th thing you need to know…..............................110

28th thing you need to know…..............................111

Chapter 4: Pharmacological Properties 112

29th thing you need to know…..............................112

Strong Sensory Stimulant & Soothing Sedative States 113

30th thing you need to know..............................113

31st thing you need to know... 113

32nd thing you need to know... 114

Definitive Doses..114

33rd thing you need to know..............................114

34th thing you need to know..............................115

35th thing you need to know..............................116

36th thing you need to know..............................120

Satisfy Sensitivities & Thwart Tolerances: Proper Practices 120

37th thing you need to know..............................120

38th thing you need to know..............................120

39th thing you need to know..............................121

40th thing you need to know..............................121

41st thing you need to know... 121

42nd thing you need to know... 122

43rd thing you need to know..............................123

44th thing you need to know..............................123

45th thing you need to know..............................124

Efficacious Effectivity 125

46th thing you need to know..............................125

47th thing you need to know...............................125

48th thing you need to know...............................125

49th thing you need to know...............................125

50th thing you need to know...............................126

Current Costs 126

51st thing you need to know... 126

52nd thing you need to know... 126

53rd thing you need to know................................127

54th thing you need to know................................128

Chapter 5: Bonuses & Benefits 129

Inflammatory Illnesses Inhibitor 129

55th thing you need to know................................129

Traditional Therapies & Treatments....................130

56th thing you need to know................................130

57th thing you need to know................................131

58th thing you need to know................................131

59th thing you need to know................................132

60th thing you need to know................................132

61st thing you need to know... 133

62nd thing you need to know... 133

63rd thing you need to know................................133

64th thing you need to know................................134

65th thing you need to know………………………….134

66th thing you need to know………………………….134

67th thing you need to know………………………….135

68th thing you need to know………………………….135

69th thing you need to know………………………….136

Chapter 6: Prudent & Precautionary Practices…..137

Misuse Measures ……………………………………………137

70th thing you need to know………………………….137

71st thing you need to know… …………………….137

72nd thing you need to know… …………………….138

73rd thing you need to know………………………….138

74th thing you need to know………………………….138

75th thing you need to know………………………….139

Critical Concerns & Conditions …………………….139

76th thing you need to know………………………….140

77th thing you need to know………………………….140

Safeness & Sustainability ………………………………141

78th thing you need to know………………………….141

79th thing you need to know………………………….141

Toxicological Truths …………………………………….142

80th thing you need to know………………………….142

81st thing you need to know… …………………….143

Strength Sports 143

82nd thing you need to know… 143

Chapter 7: Aftereffects Assessments 145

Chronic Consumers' Conditions...........................145

83rd thing you need to know…............................145

Addictive Aspects 146

84th thing you need to know…............................146

Digestive Damage & Liver Liabilities....................147

85th thing you need to know…............................147

Psychological Problems.......................................147

86th thing you need to know…............................147

Waging Withdrawals...148

87th thing you need to know…............................148

88th thing you need to know…............................148

89th thing you need to know…............................149

Chapter 8: Legalities & Liabilities 150

90th thing you need to know….............................150

91st thing you need to know… 150

92nd thing you need to know… 150

93rd thing you need to know…............................151

94th thing you need to know…............................151

95th thing you need to know…............................151

96th thing you need to know……………………….152

Social Standing …………………………………….152

97th thing you need to know……………………….152

98th thing you need to know……………………….153

99th thing you need to know……………………….153

Kratom's Kismet: Future Fate…………………154

100th thing you need to know………………………154

101st thing you need to know… ……………….155

Conclusion ……………………………………………156

CBD: 101 Things You Need To Know About CBD Oil

Introduction 1

Congratulations on downloading "*CBD: 101 Things You Need to Know About CBD Oil!*"

This book was designed to shed as much light on CBD Oil as possible. From supporting you in understanding what the supplement is and where it comes from to discovering why it is used and what side effects you may face when using it, this guide contains everything. It truly is the most comprehensive guide on the market to support you in understanding CBD Oil and how it can positively benefit you or your loved ones who are considering using it.

CBD Oil has been recognized and studied since it was discovered more than half a century ago. In that time, researchers have discovered fascinating information about this supplement and what it can do for our health. If you are ready to learn all about the supplement that everyone is talking about, this book is exactly the right place to be. You are going to learn all that there is to know.

One important thing when it comes to our health

is recognizing that being well-informed is necessary. With supplements such as CBD Oil, which is still illegal in many places, the information shared online and in the media can be highly controversial. Many are still morally against it based on the nature of its origin, whereas, other more liberal people are extremely excited by it and the many things it can do for us and our health.

Educating yourself and making sure that you are well-informed about the truth can support you in making a choice that works for *your* health. Remember, what goes into your body needs to be right for *you*. So, stay informed and make the best choice for yourself.

Now, if you are ready to get informed, get ready to be impressed! You will not find anything as comprehensive as this online, all in one place. This is the perfect book to support beginners in educating themselves on the values of this supplement and how it works. If you are ready to learn more, begin! And of course, enjoy!

Chapter 1: What is CBD Oil?

These are the essential facts you need to know about what CBD oil is and where it comes from. These facts will help you understand the history of CBD oil, what part of the plant it is extracted from, and how this contributes to the plant working on your body.

What is CBD Oil?

1st thing you need know...

CBD is one of at least 113 unique cannabinoid chemical compounds found in Cannabis and Hemp Plants. This list is not believed to be exhausted as scientists are regularly discovering new cannabinoid chemical compounds on regular basis. Many of these compounds are either irrelevant or are still being researched so that they can be applied in modern and alternative medicine.

2nd thing you need know...

Although CBD is found in Cannabis plants, THC is the most common and abundantly found cannabinoid present in Cannabis. In reverse, THC is found only in trace amounts in Hemp plants whereas CBD is the dominant, naturally occurring component.

3rd thing you need know...

Cannabidiol is known to account for up to 40% of the extracts derived from the Hemp plant. Other extracts include Hemp Oil and Hemp Seed Oil, each of which is used for different purposes.

Hemp Seed Oil is well known for having a healthy fatty acid profile which promotes healing. This means that Hemp Seed Oil is often used for treating inflammation and is good for various skin conditions such as eczema. Whereas, Hemp Oil is still typically used for CBD Oil.

4th thing you need know...

Despite being a relative of THC, the compound in marijuana that gets you high, CBD is not an addictive compound.

Unlike THC, CBD interacts naturally with our internal systems without being psychotropic, meaning it doesn't get you high. This important biochemical feature of CBD makes it a safer treatment option than medical Marijuana.

5th thing you need know...

CBD is classified as a "food supplement" in many countries. This means that when taking it, you are not actually ingesting a form of what is considered to be a drug, but rather, you are taking a natural supplement.

CBD has many great medical benefits, which I will discuss in *"Chapter 2: Why Should I Use CBD Oil?"*

Where Does it Come From?

6th thing you need know...

In recent years CBD has gained in popularity due to its many benefits such as relief from chronic pain and ailments such as seizure disorders.

7th thing you need know...

Despite not being able to get you high, CBD Oil will cause significant changes in your body. These changes are caused by the cannabinoids attaching themselves to your endocannabinoid system, allowing them to regulate functions which support relief from pain and other difficult or debilitating symptoms.

8th thing you need know...

Hemp is the least processed form of a Cannabis plant. It also happens to be the plant that contains the highest volume of CBD that can be extracted and used for medical benefits such as anxiety, epilepsy, nausea and cancer.

9th thing you need know...

Despite both coming from the Cannabis Sativa plant, Hemp and Marijuana are two very different things. They both have different genetics based on being different strains of the same plant. Also, they are cultivated for different uses.

Historically, and due to historical laws, Hemp was a legal crop that could be grown for the creation of fibers such as cloth and paper. Marijuana, however, has been outlawed in most countries for quite some time and is not typically used for anything beyond its psychoactive effects.

10th thing you need know...

Marijuana farmers have spent a long time selectively breeding Marijuana strains to increase THC levels in their plants. Hemp farmers, on the other hand, have barely altered the plant at all. This means that these plants are still incredibly high in CBD Oil, hence why most CBD Oil comes from hemp farmers.

11*th* *thing you need know...*

CBD Oil is present in Hemp Oil but not in Hemp *Seed* Oil. The CBD Oil that is generally consumed, however, is an entirely separate extract all on its own.

CBD Oil that is extracted to be used as a health supplement is extracted in a manner that allows it to stay pure and free of THC and other radicals that may take away from the quality of the oil itself.

12*th* *thing you need know...*

The way CBD Oil is extracted from the plant is crucial in ensuring the quality of the oil is kept in tact. When not extracted efficiently, CBD Oil will be inferior, and therefore will not have as great of an impact on supporting individuals in experiencing the health benefits. The correct way to extract CBD Oil is by the way of carbon dioxide (CO_2) to maintain its integrity.

What is A Cannabinoid?

13th thing you need know...

A Cannabinoid is known to be the primary chemical compound that was discovered in the Hemp and Cannabis plants.

14th thing you need know...

Cannabinoids were discovered in the 1940s with scientists originally discovering CBD and CBN in the trichomes of the Hemp plant. THC was not discovered until much later in 1964. Scientists have continued to research the plant for the past seventy plus years, finding approximately 111 more cannabinoids since.

Chapter 2: Why Should I Use CBD Oil?

This chapter is going to tell you all of the reasons why you would want to use CBD Oil. This oil was derived for the benefit of its medicinal values, so everything you learn in this chapter will highlight these benefits, and support you in understanding how valuable this oil truly is.

Why is CBD Oil Good For You?

15th thing you need know...

Unlike other medicines that are commonly prescribed for the same uses, CBD Oil has nothing in it that will make you feel "high".

Many conventional medicines prescribed for the same purpose that CBD Oil can be used for, often produce a high feeling, or otherwise, alter the personality and state of the individual in a way that may make them feel like they are distant from themselves.

CBD Oil, however, will not create any of these effects. It works within your body without having any psychoactive impact on you.

16th *thing you need know...*

CBD Oil is considered to be good for you because it is a whole plant medicine. Whole plant medicines have continued to grow in popularity over the years, assisting individuals in choosing safer alternatives to conventional medicines.

Additionally, because they are whole plants without any additives, they are believed to be easier and safer for the body to digest and use without producing negative side effects.

17th *thing you need know...*

Many conventional medicines prescribed for the same reasons as CBD Oil are known to have a long list of unhealthy side effects. Many of these often include the side effect of "death."

CBD Oil contains very few side effects. However, the side effects which can occur through using CBD Oil will be discussed in *"Chapter 5: Side effects of CBD Oil."*

18th *thing you need know...*

CBD Oil is known to promote emotional homeostasis. This is a state whereby users minimize the ups and downs that are often incurred by emotional upsets, which are known to be common in many ailments, including anything from as simple as chronic pain to as drastic as a terminal illness.

Taking a supplement that can support your well-being while also promote your emotional homeostasis means that you will experience less stress. When you experience less stress, not only do you feel better emotionally, but your body also has a stronger chance to fight against anything that may be ailing it. Stress in itself can be an illness. So, no longer having to face these stressors can have a major positive impact on your overall health.

19th thing you need know...

If you are interested in the environment and want to support your own health in the process, CBD Oil is a great choice.

CBD Oil is a highly sustainable product, which as mentioned previously is derived from a plant that has many uses. That means that the same plant that was grown to produce your medicine is also being used to create fibers to be used in sustainable and ethical cloth and paper products. This also means that fewer crops have to be grown and the crops are less damaging to the environment.

20th thing you need know...

Hemp plants are ready to be harvested much quicker than other medicines. It is easier to produce higher amounts of Hemp plants from smaller crop fields.

21st thing you need know...

CBD Oil is known to be an antioxidant, meaning that it can support your body in eliminating free radicals.

Free radicals in the body have been known to promote the onset of many diseases and ailments, such as cancer. Eliminating them is great for supporting your overall long-term health and preventing these diseases from having the capacity to develop in your system.

22nd thing you need know...

Because of its nature, CBD Oil has the capacity to treat many things. This means that while you may be taking it for one specific reason, it will also be working on other symptoms within your body. So, while you experience relief from your primary concern, you will also experience greater health in other areas as a result of this medicine.

It is one of the few medicines you can take that will have many positive benefits, as opposed to strictly treating the specific condition you are focused on.

23rd thing you need know...

Unlike many conventional medicines, CBD Oil can be taken in many different ways. As a result, you can easily get it into your system in whatever way works best for you. This versatility makes it excellent for treating many ailments because you can get it directly to the source of the symptom quickly and in the most effective way possible in a way that is also more comfortable for you.

24th thing you need know...

Instead of reaching for over-the-counter medicines like ibuprofen and acetaminophen, many clinicians believe that the future includes CBD Oil being used as a standard-practice supplement in everyone's cupboards. The aforementioned medicines, when ingested too frequently, have been shown to deteriorate the stomach lining and increase problematic symptoms such as heartburn and acid reflux.

Using CBD Oil as an alternative would likely prove to be safer and more effective for those who need relief from symptoms such as headaches or general muscle aches and pains.

25th thing you need know...

CBD Oil has been known to counteract the impacts of THC. This is why many recreational marijuana growers will minimize CBD content while maximizing THC content. It allows people to experience greater psychoactive effects. This is also why having 0.3% or less THC in your CBD Oil is not a bad thing. The CBD will counteract it and prevent you from experiencing psychoactive effects.

Is it Safe?

26th thing you need know...

Although CBD Oil is praised for being highly natural, some individuals may not be able to take it due to it poorly interacting with other medicines that they may already be taking.

There may be other health-related issues that reduce the safeness of CBD Oil, so it is always a good idea to talk to your healthcare practitioner before ingesting any prescribed supplement.

If you are with a practitioner who tends to have conservative views, they may immediately rule out CBD Oil simply because they do not believe in using it at all. If this is the case, you may benefit from going to a doctor who is CBD-informed and able to genuinely support you in making a choice that is right for you, versus making a choice that is based on your healthcare practitioner's morals.

27th thing you need know...

CBD Oil is a natural plant extract. In its purest form it can be unsafe for your body. This is why those who sell CBD Oil will dilute it with carrier oils such as fractionated coconut oil or jojoba oil. It can then be safely applied or ingested without producing negative or harmful side effects to you. When buying CBD Oil, ensure that you thoroughly research how the oil has been extracted and what carrier oils have been used, as this can also affect the quality of the oil.

It is important that you never apply pure CBD Oil to your body or ingest it, as it may cause severe damage. All natural plant extracts, including standard essential oils such as peppermint oil or eucalyptus oil, are extremely strong and can cause irritation, burns, or other damage to any part of the body that it may come into contact with.

28th thing you need know...

Some medicines are known to have side effects that can actually enhance the symptom that the user is attempting to avoid. For example, some anti-depressants are known to increase symptoms of depression and the tendency of experiencing suicidal thoughts, thus putting the user at a greater risk of suicide.

CBD Oil, on the other hand, does not have any side effects like this. Typically, the worst side effect is that it will not work or that you need your dosage adjusted.

Therefore, using CBD Oil may be safer because it reduces the risk of facing challenging side effects that may be detrimental or fatal to the user.

29th thing you need know...

Although it cannot combine with all medicines, most medicines are not impacted by the use of CBD Oil. This means, you can use CBD Oil as a safe alternative to pain medications to help you alleviate symptoms that you may experience from other medical treatments.

This has been especially popular amongst cancer patients who may be experiencing negative symptoms and side effects from harsh cancer treatments such as radiation. Taking CBD Oil can minimize these symptoms while allowing the radiation to successfully complete what it was put in the body to do.

30th thing you need know...

CBD Oil is believed to have neuroprotective properties, meaning that it can support and protect the neurological system. To those who are struggling with neurological conditions such as seizures or multiple sclerosis, CBD Oil can provide great relief from the symptoms of these conditions.

31st thing you need know...

CBD Oil is believed to have a positive impact on the circulatory system. When taken in the correct dosage, it can lower high blood pressure and promote a healthier functioning heart. It is likely that the stress- and anxiety-reducing properties of the oil are responsible for lowering blood pressure.

Common Uses

32nd thing you need know...

CBD Oil is known to fight against cancer. CBD and other cannabinoids found in the Cannabis plant have been proven to have an anti-tumor effect, and are also known to support the fight with standard treatments.

In a recent study, CBD was successful in stopping multiple different cervical cancer cells in a patient. It has also increased tumor cell death in both colon cancer and leukemia. It is also known to be promising in combination therapies that many medics use for breast and prostate cancers.

Combination therapy means that it can be used alongside other conventional or alternative therapies, working together to promote the reversal of tumors and cancer cells in patients who have been diagnosed with varying types of cancer.

33rd thing you need know...

Many people use CBD Oil due to the fact that this oil is incredible for relieving pain. This analgesic (a supplement with pain-relieving effects) interacts with receptors in your brain and immune system to support your body in alleviating pain and reducing any inflammation that may be contributing to the pain. Due to the nature of this supplement, these benefits are often experienced with zero side effects.

34th thing you need know...

One of the most incredible and notable features of CBD Oil is its ability to minimize and eliminate seizures from patients who were previously experiencing many.

Some producers and distributors of CBD Oil have noted that they have witnessed patients, who experienced more than 100 seizures a day, have absolutely none for several weeks on end after using CBD Oil.

The oil has even been noted to stop a seizure from happening within minutes of symptoms beginning.

35th thing you need know...

Anxiety is something that a large portion of the population faces. The Anxiety and Depression Association of America (ADAA) estimates that more than 40 million Americans who are over the age of 18 are impacted or affected by anxiety. This accounts for approximately 18% of the entire American population.

CBD Oil has shown promising effects in minimizing and eliminating anxiety disorder, even for those experiencing crippling anxiety that prevents them from leading a typical lifestyle with basic activities.

CBD Oil works on anxiety by relaxing an individual in their limbic and paralimbic brain areas. Again, CBD Oil can stunt the effects of a panic or anxiety attack within minutes of an individual consuming the oil.

36th thing you need know...

A lesser-known benefit of CBD Oil is that it is capable of supporting individuals in reducing their risk of developing diabetes.

Recently, Neuropharmacology released a study that showed that CBD Oil prevented 67% of non-obese diabetes-prone female mice from developing the disease, whereas, 100% of untreated mice with the same likelihood of developing the disease did go on to develop the disease.

There are still studies being done to show how effective this is for adult humans, though the results are looking very promising.

37th *thing you need know...*

Many individuals in modern society face a wide range of sleep-related issues. From experiencing restless sleep that results in them waking feeling un-rested to full-blown insomnia.

One of the "side effects" of CBD Oil is promoting a better rest in adults, sometimes leading them to feel sleepy after taking the supplement. This means that instead of using addictive and potentially damaging medicines that can cause false positive sleep patterns, you can use a safe alternative through this holistic supplement. CBD Oil has been found to promote a healthier and sounder sleep pattern without creating any addictions or harming you in any way.

38th *thing you need know...*

One interesting benefit many users claim to gain from CBD Oil is that this supplement reduces acne.

Acne is believed to develop in individuals for

many reasons, ranging from genetics to bacteria or even underlying conditions.

Science has recently shown that using CBD Oil through topical application has the potential to improve acne conditions, likely as a result of its anti-inflammatory effects. So, using CBD Oil can help reduce and reverse problematic anxiety in individuals who may be struggling to keep their face clear and free of acne.

39th thing you need know...

CBD Oil has shown to have antipsychotic properties. While it is not yet being issued in standard practice, many studies have shown that CBD Oil has the capacity to minimize psychotic episodes, such as those linked to schizophrenia or other mental disorders that produce psychotic symptoms.

Using this supplement has shown promising benefits in reducing psychotic symptoms and episodes, supporting those who have been diagnosed with these types of mental disorders in their ability to lead a higher quality life, free of challenging and problematic symptoms that can prevent them from living a typical life.

40th thing you need know...

Many addictions therapists have been using CBD Oil as a way to help individuals who are quitting hard drugs such as heroin and methamphetamine to reduce difficult symptoms of withdrawal.

In studies that have been done to investigate the successful benefits of this medicine, researchers have shown that CBD Oil can support drug-addicted individuals in reducing difficult symptoms as well as in preventing dependency and drug-seeking behaviors. In other words, those who were using CBD Oil as a part of their treatment were able to go several days, or longer, without actively seeking out drugs to support their addiction.

41st thing you need know...

Quitting smoking is another great benefit of using CBD Oil. Much like with supporting individuals in quitting their addictions to harder drugs, CBD Oil can also support individuals in quitting their addiction to cigarettes.

Research studies showed that those who used placebo inhalers experienced no change in their overall cigarette consumption, whereas, those who used CBD Oil smoked nearly 40% fewer cigarettes on average each day.

42ⁿᵈ *thing you need know...*

Fibromyalgia is a chronic pain condition that has no known cause and few tried and true remedies that work for everyone who takes them. It is a fairly mysterious condition that cannot be treated by others.

CBD Oil has been shown to be a powerful pain remedy and symptom remedy for those diagnosed with fibromyalgia. In studies that have been done, virtually everyone who was put on the CBD Oil treatment saw significantly reduced symptoms, with some of them even going on to live symptom-free.

43ʳᵈ *thing you need know...*

Post Traumatic Stress Disorder (PTSD) is a highly complex form of advanced anxiety that is experienced by those who have been in traumatic situations. Many think of post-war veterans when they think of PTSD, but the reality is that this disorder actually impacts far more than just them.

Those who have been exposed to varying degrees of abuse throughout their life have also been shown to develop PTSD as a result as well. In these individuals, using CBD Oil has shown to have a profound impact on supporting them in living symptom-free.

Those who take it have been shown to experience great relief, thus making it a great potential treatment for those living with PTSD. Due to the anti-anxiety, anti-stress, anti-inflammatory, and antipsychotic effects of CBD Oil, it supports those living with PTSD in experiencing a more mentally stable environment for them.

44th thing you need know...

Research and studies have also been done with those who have been living with either Crohn's disease or irritable bowel syndrome (IBS).

Scientists have discovered that CBD Oil may have a powerful impact on supporting the relief of symptoms related to these two conditions.

Due to its anti-inflammatory properties and the way CBD Oil interacts with the part of your body responsible for controlling gut function, CBD Oil has been shown to support individuals with either of these conditions in being able to pass bowel movements with greater ease and less symptomatic pain and/or suffering.

45th thing you need know...

Multiple Sclerosis is a disease that is chronic and progressive. It damages nerves in your brain and spinal cord, leading to the loss of use of many muscles and body parts. Those with this disease are known to have difficulty speaking and using muscular coordination. They also struggle with blurred vision and severe fatigue as a result of the disease.

Studies have shown that using CBD Oil can greatly improve symptoms relating to this disease, potentially even reversing the symptoms and protecting the body against multiple sclerosis altogether. Using CBD Oil may help those with multiple sclerosis regain control over their muscles and live a better life following treatment than they would have without the use of CBD Oil.

46th thing you need know...

Rheumatoid arthritis is a painful form of arthritis that damages bones and joints and can lead to a malformed body over time.

Due to CBD Oil having anti-inflammatory effects and inflammation is one of the leading symptoms and causes of degeneration with rheumatoid arthritis, taking this oil may support those living with this condition to experience reduced symptoms.

It has been shown to decrease joint destruction and slow down disease progression, allowing those with a diagnosis of rheumatoid arthritis to lead a longer, happier, and healthier life.

47th *thing you need know...*

Although the research into this one is not as extensive, studies have shown that individuals who are suffering from broken bones have healed faster with the use of CBD Oil than without.

Bone growth is considered to be one of the benefits of this supplement. Studies are continuing to be done to see if this supplement can support individuals in having improved bone health overall, potentially contributing to faster broken bones healing as well as fewer symptomatic side effects of osteoporosis.

48th *thing you need know...*

Psoriasis is a painful and uncomfortable skin condition that results in the extremely dry flaky skin on those who suffer with it.

When used topically in an ointment, cream,

serum, or lotion, CBD Oil has been shown to support individuals in minimizing their symptoms of psoriasis and experiencing greater skin health. Since this condition can be itchy, painful, and embarrassing, it is extremely helpful to those suffering to experience freedom from their problematic symptoms.

49*th* thing you need know...

Dyskinesia and Restless Leg Syndrome (RLS) are two conditions that cause an involuntary muscle movement in those who are struggling with the conditions.

CBD, when combined with a TRPV-1 blocker, has been shown to reduce symptoms of these conditions, supporting individuals in minimizing involuntary muscle movement and thus having greater control over their muscles in general.

50*th* thing you need know...

Due to our poor diets and the way we live our lives; many of us live with some form of a gastrointestinal disease that can cause nausea and vomiting, as well as decreased appetite.

CBD Oil has been shown to relieve these symptoms and support individuals struggling with poor gut health in experiencing an increased appetite so they can nourish their bodies with ease.

As a side note, THC has also been a proven effective method in supporting the same benefits. In fact, some clinics will prescribe "dronabinol", which is a medicine made with THC, to those who are suffering. However, clinics are showing that CBD has greater promise in supporting good health over THC as it contains fewer side effects which can affect the patient.

51st thing you need know...

In people who have injuries to their spinal cord, CBD Oil is great in helping to treat both the nerve damage and the symptomatic pain experienced by this injury.

For those who have suffered from traumatic accidents, this may be revolutionary in providing non-addictive pain relief to victims.

52nd thing you need know...

CBD Oil is in the process of being studied to understand how it may help individuals who have experienced a stroke.

The oil has shown to be effective in studies where symptoms of a stroke, such as nerve damage, is being treated and reversed with the use of CBD Oil.

While this is still in the very early stages of research, the findings have been promising in showing that individuals are regaining painless use of their limbs and muscles with CBD Oil treatment following a stroke.

Chapter 3: How Do I Take CBD Oil?

Taking CBD Oil clearly has many benefits and positive outcomes for those who use it. However, you may still be wondering *how* to use it. One incredible thing about this supplement is that it is extremely versatile in how you can take it and how much you can take of it. Typically, the way CBD Oil is used depends on what type of ailment you are treating. Here are some facts that you should know about on how you can use CBD Oil.

Topically

53rd thing you need know…

Because it is a natural plant extract, pure CBD Oil should never be taken topically without first being diluted into some form of tincture, lotion, balm, or otherwise. Pure CBD Oil applied directly to the skin may cause irritation, taking away from the healing benefits that it is otherwise known for having.

54th thing you need know…

Most distributors of CBD Oil will have a variety of different topical CBD Oil products that you can use. These products are made differently so that they target different purposes as well as with varying dosages.

It is always a good idea to seek support in discovering which one will work best for your needs unless you are already educated on what exactly you are looking for.

55th thing you need know...

Topical CBD Oil products do not have the same affect that the ingestible CBD Oil products do. This means that they are faster working and that you get a more focused healing benefit for your desired symptom. For example, if you have psoriasis, applying CBD Oil topically will work directly on psoriasis, whereas, ingesting it would work on your entire body and take significantly longer to improve your psoriasis.

56th thing you need know...

Applying CBD Oil topically is the least invasive method for using CBD Oil.

Both ingesting it and inhaling it will work directly on your entire body, whereas applying it topically focuses primarily on the issue it has been applied to.

Furthermore, because CBD Oil in topical products interacts with the CB2 receptors near your skin, they activate the endocannabinoid system. This means that unlike other varieties of topical treatments, CBD Oil will never actually enter your bloodstream through topical products.

57th *thing you need know...*

Most topical products will advise you to "apply liberally" because human skin is known to have a low absorption rate for cannabinoids. While this works great to prevent it from entering the bloodstream, it also means that you need to use a lot in order for the skin to actually absorb enough of the product for it to be beneficial.

58th *thing you need know...*

Topical CBD products are not just used on skin-related issues. They are also used on joint-related issues and acute pain, such as with rheumatoid arthritis or fibromyalgia. Applying it directly to the pain itself can cause quicker relief, making it more effective for some of these symptoms than actually ingesting the CBD Oil.

59th *thing you need know...*

Some chronic conditions, such as fibromyalgia, will use CBD Oil through ingestible products to maintain ongoing symptom relief as well as use topical treatments to work directly on symptoms that may flare up despite the ongoing use of CBD Oil supplements.

This supports individuals in experiencing nearly total symptom relief. This combination treatment may be used on a variety of conditions that cause pain or other acute physical symptoms.

Ingested

60th thing you need know...

Ingesting CBD Oil tends to be one of the easiest ways for beginners or children to take CBD oil for their symptoms. This is the most commonly prescribed method for those who are using CBD Oil to treat a condition.

When you swallow a CBD oil pill, you are swallowing concentrated oil that is then passed through the digestive system and metabolized by the liver. This allows it to enter into your bloodstream where it begins to work on your symptoms. This is the same way most daily vitamins are delivered into your system.

61st *thing you need know...*

Because the process of ingesting oil requires the capsule to first be passed through the digestive system, ingesting oil can take up to two hours before full effects are experienced. However, many people report experiencing positive effects from it within minutes of taking the capsule.

This means that ingesting CBD Oil through a concentrated capsule form can have slow-release type effects on users, allowing them to experience symptom relief for up to four hours after taking a single dosage.

62nd *thing you need know...*

If you prefer not to swallow a capsule, CBD Oil can also come in a small pill that you place under your tongue and melt with your saliva. This allows the oil to enter directly into your bloodstream, giving you quicker symptom relief lasting for several hours.

For people with random and quick onset of symptoms, this can be a great way for quickly alleviating those symptoms without having to wait for the digestive system to break down the capsule and digest the oil.

63rd thing you need know...

Another way that many people ingest CBD Oil is through eating what dispensaries often call "gourmet treats."

These are baked goods which are made with CBD Oil to deliver the same results through digestion but in a way that eliminates the swallowing of a capsule or the need to melt a pill under your tongue.

For some people, eating smaller rations of food made with CBD Oil throughout the day can allow the oil to continually deliver consistent results all day long. Some foods that are regularly made with CBD Oil include varieties of yogurt, popcorn, and cooking oil that can be mixed into salad dressing recipes or used as finishing oil for various dishes, butter, coffee, smoothies or pasta sauce.

There are many varieties of edibles these days. You can find anything that works best for you and consume that to receive the great benefits of CBD Oil without having to take it in pill form.

64th *thing you need know...*

If you are taking CBD Oil in capsule form, the dosage can easily be adjusted by the dispensary. This means that you can request lower dosage and higher dosage CBD Oil capsules that allow you to receive your best results from the supplement without feeling like you are overdoing it.

These can be considered akin to "regular strength" and "extra strength" supplements for those who are using them this way.

65th *thing you need know...*

Other forms of CBD Oil that are not edibles but are not capsules either include tinctures and concentrates. These are unique creations with CBD Oil that are taken orally and allow the CBD Oil to almost immediately enter the endocannabinoid system in the body so that you begin to experience immediate effects.

Tinctures are great because they can be flavored, making it more enjoyable to take. Concentrates can be used for higher dosages and quick-relief from symptoms.

Vaporized

66th *thing you need know...*

CBD oil can be vaporized, which is one of the leading reasons why many people may confuse it for THC or Marijuana and fall under the false belief that it can make you "high."

As you already know from Chapter 1, there are key differences between CBD Oil and Marijuana or THC Oil. Vaporizing CBD Oil will not deliver any form of high unless the oil has THC in it. When you vaporize CBD Oil, you are still taking the same thing. You are simply delivering it to your system by a different means.

67th *thing you need know...*

Vaporizing CBD Oil was one of the first methods for taking CBD Oil before it was researched in depth and new ways were discovered.

Researchers later looked at the plant and searched for new ways that they could isolate the CBD Oil compound and create other methods for taking the supplement that did not involve vaporizing.

68th *thing you need know...*

Many people prefer to vaporize CBD Oil because it enters the lungs and then immediately enters the bloodstream along with your oxygen. This results in quick relief from symptoms which may not experience relief from topical treatments and may take too long to relieve through ingesting it.

69th thing you need know...

Vaporizing is not the same as smoking. When you vaporize something, enough heat is being applied to it that it essentially becomes a steam. The CBD compound is then transported into your body through this steam.

When you smoke something, you burn it to the point that it is smoking and it enters your body through the smoke. While smoke has been shown to have carcinogenic effects, vapor has not. This means that vaporizing CBD Oil refrains from burning off some of it and wasting it, as well as prevents you from experiencing adverse side effects of the smoke.

People who have chronic asthma or lung conditions will often vaporize CBD Oil for instant relief and no adverse side effects that may come from smoking.

70th thing you need know...

Vaporizing CBD Oil requires you to use a pure

form of CBD Oil concentrate. This is the kind that you may ingest, but that you typically do not want to apply directly to your skin.

You want to make sure you are using pure CBD Oil because you do not want to be vaporizing and inhaling any other ingredients that may be harmful to your health.

If you plan on vaporizing, make sure your dispensary knows this, so that they can administer the proper form of oil to you, so that you do not experience any harmful or adverse reactions.

71st thing you need know...

Vaporizers come in many shapes and sizes. You can purchase pen-style vaporizers that are small and easy to transport, portable vaporizers that are larger but still easy to transport, and desktop or stationary vaporizers that are much larger and tend to deliver higher dosages with a plug-in feature that will vaporize the oil for you.

These vaporizers may deliver you the vapor via a tube, a bag or a balloon, or as a direct draw vaporizer. They tend to be heated with conduction, convection, or infrared heating systems that are designed to control the output temperature so as to heat your oil just enough to be vaporized but not so much to be burnt and turned into a smoke.

72nd thing you need know...

Some vaporizers are made in a way that allows them to vaporize dry herbs. This means that your dispensary may distribute a piece of the cannabis plant that is high in CBD content but features little to no THC content.

Remember, in order for these supplements to be legal, they must have less than 0.3% THC in them. This means that if your distributor gives you something like this, you are still not going to get high from the herb.

However, it is still important to communicate with your distributor as some do carry herbs that are high in THC as well for other medicinal values.

73rd thing you need know...

Despite other delivery systems becoming available, many believe that vaporizing should still be the most commonly used form for delivering CBD Oil to a patient's system. This is because topical creams require a high amount of product in order to be effective, and ingested CBD Oil can take longer to activate.

Furthermore, using a vaporizer is much safer than smoking the herb, thus making it the safest and most effective method for delivering the CBD into your body.

Chapter 4: Who Should Take CBD Oil?

In this chapter, we are going to discover facts about who can safely take CBD Oil and who cannot. Naturally, you want to make sure that you are safe to take it to refrain from experiencing any negative side effects. This is simply common knowledge when planning on taking any new supplements or medicinal products!

General Facts

74th thing you need know...

Based on research, the majority of individuals can take CBD Oil and not face risks of having any major side effects as a result of taking the supplement.

This is one of the safest and most versatile supplements on the market that can support a variety of medicinal causes without causing adverse side effects to various age groups.

75th thing you need know...

In addition to humans being able to take CBD Oil, veterinarians and researchers have begun to realize that CBD Oil can also be used by animals for many causes.

In particular, dogs with epilepsy or senior dogs with arthritis have been shown to have great positive reactions to the supplement. It has also been tested for a number of other ailments in animals and has shown to have the same positive effect.

It is important to note, however, that using other forms of cannabis including marijuana is not safe for animals so refrain from using anything without the support or assistance of your vet.

Also, how animals take the oil should be monitored to refrain from giving it to them in a way that may be harmful. In this case, the method of delivery would be harmful and not the supplement itself.

Children

76th thing you need know...

Because THC and CBD are not the same, many children can safely take CBD supplements without experiencing any adverse reactions.

Frequently, CBD Oil is used to treat conditions such as chronic pain conditions and epilepsy in children.

77th thing you need know...

Not all CBD Oil is made the same. For this reason, you need to ensure that you are getting your CBD over-the-counter from a trusted dispensary.

CBD Oil that you purchase online may have some degree of THC in it which is not recommended or advised for consumption by children. While CBD will not create any psychoactive symptoms, THC will if it is present in larger amounts and this can be dangerous for children.

Although the FDA does work hard to eliminate any untrustworthy online dealers who may be selling CBD Oil with higher-than-allowed levels of THC in it, it does not mean that every seller will be properly screened and shut down if necessary.

It is advised that you take all necessary precautions, especially with children, to refrain them from having any adverse reactions.

78th thing you need know...

Especially with children, consulting with a trained healthcare professional is important.

While CBD Oil itself is relatively safe and has no instances of death or serious lasting side effects, giving it to young children may not always be safe.

Some doctors may advise against it and instead offer other therapies. That being said, always take the time to make sure you understand your doctor's overall stance on CBD Oil.

Many conservative doctors are still morally against it and therefore will suggest that absolutely no one should be using this supplement. Working together with a CBD-informed healthcare professional can support you in making the right choice.

79th thing you need know...

Children who live with Autism, Sensory Processing Disorder (SPD,) ADD or ADHD or other disorders that are especially challenging in youth, having a CBD supplement can help manage symptoms and support the child in feeling more capable of "fitting in" to their environment.

CBD Oil has been shown to minimize the stress that the child may face and support them in feeling a sense of belonging in their environment.

80th thing you need know...

Currently, CBD Oil is not legal in every state. For that reason, you need to be careful to look over state laws and only purchase when it is legal for your state.

Taking the oil as a consenting adult in a state where it is illegal can be incriminating, never mind giving the supplement to a youth.

Make sure that you know the laws and that you follow them accordingly to refrain from being incriminated for using this supplement.

Adults

81st thing you need know...

CBD Oil is not necessarily the cheapest medication available, though you can find places that will make it more affordable.

Most healthcare insurance will not cover the purchase, so you will need to purchase CBD Oil out of your own pocket. That being said, there are some programs that certain dispensaries are enrolled in where you can enroll to make the supplement cheaper for you to purchase.

82nd thing you need know...

Just like with children, adults who are considering using CBD Oil need to consult a healthcare practitioner.

While CBD Oil in itself is not dangerous, having a trained professional supporting you in finding the right way to deliver it into your system and how much to take is important.

Someone who knows what they are doing will support you in using enough that you can feel the positive effects without overdoing it and wasting your money or risking your health.

Seniors

83rd *thing you need know...*

In seniors who are facing common symptoms of aging, such as arthritis and other pain-related symptoms, using CBD Oil is considered to be a safer alternative to having other medicines available for these conditions.

CBD Oil can provide the same degree of symptom relief without other adverse reactions that may, in some cases, be even harsher to seniors.

84th *thing you need know...*

Seniors tend to be more at risk for developing diseases such as Alzheimer's and Parkinson's disease. Due to the nature of CBD Oil being anti-inflammatory, having neuroprotective properties, and being able to calm and regulate muscle function to prevent involuntary movement, CBD Oil has proven effective in helping to relieve symptoms related to these conditions.

In the past, these conditions have caused severe discomfort and inconveniences to the individuals suffering from them, so having effective relief that could restore their quality of life is important.

85th *thing you need know...*

Later in life, many seniors find themselves being faced with a medicine cabinet that is filled with a variety of different medications. Each one of those medications often comes with their own long-list of potential side effects.

Since the older bodies of seniors are more vulnerable, they are at higher risk of facing these side effects. Many seniors even have medicines specifically prescribed to treat the symptoms of other side effects. Furthermore, not all of these medicines are covered by insurances, resulting in seniors likely having to pay enormous amounts for their medicine.

While CBD Oil is not necessarily a cheaper alternative, it may come in at around the same amount per month. Also, it is one single supplement as opposed to having many. Seniors would not have to treat for symptoms of other medicines and instead could enjoy a higher quality of life simply through the use of one single supplement, as opposed to a medicine cabinet full of them.

86th *thing you need know...*

Although CBD Oil cannot prevent death, it can

make the process of dealing with terminal illnesses a lot more bearable for those going through them.

For seniors who are regularly developing terminal illnesses having access to CBD Oil as a part of their therapy may make their elder years more enjoyable by reducing problematic symptoms and giving them the opportunity to enjoy those later years.

87th thing you need know...

Another fear that some have in later years that is not necessarily a symptom of taking medicine but more so a symptom of aging is accidentally taking a double-dosage of medicine.

Taking a supplement that has the potential to provide the same relief but is not *as dangerous* if it is taken in a double-dosage can provide a great peace of mind to seniors.

Since CBD Oil cannot produce overdoses, seniors are not at risk for accidentally taking a potentially fatal dose of medicine. Still, seniors should consult with a healthcare practitioner before using CBD Oil just to be on the side of caution.

Chapter 5: Side Effects of CBD Oil

Despite being touted for not having any problematic side effects *for most people,* CBD Oil has been reported to cause some mild, non-life threatening side effects in those who take it.

Occasionally, depending on the medical condition of those taking it, it may not be considered a safe supplement. Here are some facts that you should know about the side effects of CBD Oil.

Medicinal Considerations

88th *thing you need know...*

Those who have problems with lower blood pressure should not take CBD Oil as it can further lower blood pressure and may put them at risk of cardiac arrest.

If you have chronically low blood pressure or find yourself struggling with heart health in this way, taking CBD Oil may not be the best choice for you.

89th thing you need know...

If you are taking drugs such as steroids, calcium channel blockers, HIV antivirals, antibiotics, beta blockers, NSAIDs, oral hypoglycemic agents, or other medicines, taking CBD Oil can react with these medicines and cause negative symptoms.

It is important that if you are taking any other medicines, even temporarily, that you are transparent with your doctor about using CBD Oil and that you refrain from using the oil in combination with any medicines which may be deemed unsafe to use with CBD Oil.

90th thing you need know...

The way people metabolize CBD is vastly different, this means that people who are taking CBD Oil need to be monitored early on for symptoms to make sure that their dosage is correct.

When the dosage is correct, there should be no problematic symptoms from the CBD Oil *and* all or most of your symptoms should be minimized or alleviated.

91st thing you need know...

While some medicines work adversely with CBD Oil, some actually work well together with it. This is called combination therapy.

In order to discover whether or not CBD Oil will work well with the medications you are currently using, you should chat with a CBD-informed doctor who can support you in making an informed choice.

Symptomatic Side Effects

92nd *thing you need know...*

Despite CBD Oil being known to treat anxiety and depression, some individuals may experience increased anxiety and depression after using CBD.

While the cause for this is not entirely known, it is believed to be in relation to the fact that CBD Oil slows things down, such as your circulatory system, which may trigger symptoms of depression or anxiety in some users.

93rd *thing you need know...*

Proper CBD Oil should not have enough THC in it to react within your body. However, some individuals have shown to experience psychosis after using CBD Oil.

This may be caused by being sensitive toward the compound, or it may be because they purchased it from an untrustworthy source and it had higher than legal levels of THC in it.

It is important to make sure that you are monitored by a trained healthcare professional when using this supplement and that you are purchasing it from safe and trusted sources.

94th thing you need know...

Some individuals who take CBD Oil may find themselves experiencing nausea. In most cases, this comes from taking a higher-than-needed dosage.

For others, the concentration of the oil may be too much for their body. Switching to an alternative delivery method or choosing a different supplement or medicine altogether may be necessary for these individuals.

95th thing you need know...

In severe cases, CBD Oil may cause vomiting in individuals. Vomiting is generally caused by the body struggling to digest it or by the CBD Oil irritating the lining of the stomach.

If this is happening, avoid taking it again until you can communicate with your healthcare practitioner. It may be because you have too high of a dosage, or it may be because you are sensitive to the oil and need to choose an alternative method for relieving symptoms.

96th thing you need know...

CBD Oil is known to be great for supporting individuals in having better sleep, hence, why many use it to ward off symptoms of restless sleep or insomnia. That being said, drowsiness is known to be one of the side effects of CBD Oil.

If you are not taking it for the purpose of sleeping better at night and you feel that the drowsiness is becoming problematic, you may be able to switch your dosage or take it differently to avoid this side effect.

97th thing you need know...

Some individuals who take CBD Oil report having a dry mouth after taking it. Ingesting enough water to keep yourself healthily hydrated and sucking on cough drops or small hard candies can help keep saliva in your mouth and prevent dry mouth.

Otherwise, if it is extremely problematic, you might consider switching your dosage to avoid this symptom altogether.

98th *thing you need know...*

Some people who take CBD Oil find that they get dizzy after taking it. This may be due to having a lower blood pressure after taking the medicine.

If you experience dizziness, be sure to move slowly between lying down, sitting, and standing positions to avoid falling over. Refrain from taking any further medicine until you have communicated with your doctor. If this is a symptom of abnormally low blood pressure, continuing to take the medicine could result in harmful effects.

99th *thing you need know...*

The exact reasoning is unknown, but some individuals who use CBD Oil find themselves experiencing diarrhea afterward. This may be due to the digestive system struggling to break it down or relaxing too much.

If this happens, be sure to drink more fluids. If it persists, communicate this with your doctor and see if your dosage can be adjusted to avoid this side effect.

100th thing you need know...

Generally, people who take CBD Oil find themselves feeling an increased appetite.

Alternatively, if you are experiencing early symptoms of nausea, you may feel a decreased appetite. If you feel that your appetite has changed too much for you to maintain a healthy level of intake or like you are consistently eating too much, consider talking to your doctor to have your dosage adjusted.

101st thing you need know...

Some individuals who have Parkinson's disease have noticed increased tremors as opposed to decreased tremors when taking CBD Oil. For that reason, it may not be effective for all cases of Parkinson's disease. Still, some individuals experience great relief as a result of it.

Conclusion 1

Congratulations on reading "*CBD: 101 Things You Need to Know About CBD Oil*"!

This fun yet comprehensive guide was designed to provide you with 101 things to inform you about CBD Oil and why it is all the rage in modern culture. Everyone is talking about it, the government is legalizing it, and many are experiencing life-changing results from it. It is a seriously powerful supplement that has the power to change the way we face our health in a really positive way.

I hope that in reading this guide, you were able to get a better understanding of what CBD Oil is, where it comes from, and why it is used. I hope you were also able to learn about the pros and cons, and much more information to support you in understanding this supplement in greater detail.

Whether you are brand new to the supplement or you have been reading about it for some time, I set the intention of making this guide a one-stop source for you to learn as much as possible in one simple location.

The next step is for you to consider how CBD Oil may benefit you or the loved ones. If you find that you are leaning towards taking the supplement, communicate with a certified healthcare practitioner who is CBD-informed and who can support you in making the right choice. Always be sure to be transparent with your current health conditions and any medications you are taking as you never want to have accidental adverse reactions due to withholding the truth from your doctor.

Furthermore, make sure that you pay attention to getting your oil from a safe and trusted dispensary who knows what they are doing. Take the time to ask them how their oils are made, where they come from, and what they do to verify that they are as safe as they say they are.

You want to make sure that anything going into your body is safe for you. If they are a safe and trustworthy dispensary, they will be willing to answer any questions you have and should be happy to support you in feeling confident in your choice.

Kratom: 101 Things You Need To Know About Kratom

Introduction 2

Kratom is making a noticeable mark on both the drug industry and the medical field and bears a fast-growing reputation of being a natural wonder for its countless healthcare and wellness benefits.

Since the 19th century, Kratom has been valued in traditional medicine. However, the modern world of today is shrouding it with controversy and pressing debates. The contention gives rise to whether Kratom is a safe treatment for drug addiction or a dangerous banned substance.

Recently, Kratom plants and its products have attracted attention from various law enforcement authorities worldwide. However, with a lack of reported risk issues or fatal consequences directly arising from Kratom use, its legal use still prevails in some parts of the globe.

For those of you who are new to Kratom, it is a plant medicine that grows in some selected localities of the Southeast Asian regions, particularly in Thailand, Malaysia, Burma, and Indonesia. Its medicinal leaves are primarily effective treatments of pain symptoms and opiate addiction. It has also been reputed to be a great inhibitor of symptoms arising from a variety of anti-inflammatory diseases.

Kratom leaves contain compounds that create stimulating and sedative effects to users. According to users, Kratom produces a pleasant feeling lasting longer than a cup of coffee does. Users often also experience wakefulness, moderate euphoria and a sense of wellbeing.

Like any medicinal substances that modify mood, different dosages produce a range of effects. In general, a small amount of Kratom produces a feeling of mild stimulation and alertness, while a larger dose produces a feeling of sedation. Moderate usage of Kratom never appears to impair behaviors or promote tendencies towards violent acts.

As an opiate substitute, Kratom does not contain opiates of any kind. However, its compounds have the ability to bind to the same opiate receptors in the brain that are associated with numbing feelings, pain relief and sedation. It has been said that the effects of Kratom can exhibit similarity those of opium's mood and mind altering states.

Due to these diverse activities in the brain, Kratom produces an overall pleasing feeling. However, despite its effectiveness at curbing addiction to certain narcotics, users can then become addicted to Kratom itself.

Because of its possible nature to be an abusive drug, some agencies are in uproar over Kratom, even though it mostly enjoys a long history of safe use. The Food and Drug Administration in the US labeled Kratom as a probable dangerous drug due to its properties that can potentially harm humans. Currently, Kratom is illegal and regulated in certain countries like Thailand, Malaysia, Australia, Burma, and just recently, Ireland.

In this informative guidebook, I will present you with a compilation of 101 facts that you need to know about Kratom. These numbered and itemized details, broken down across eight chapters, will ultimately form your comprehensive understanding of Kratom and its uses.

So let us get right ahead, and find out everything you need to know about Kratom.

Chapter 1: Kratom Knowledge: A Botanical Background

Most people have differing opinions on what the term 'drug' really means. A specific drug is often different compared to its definition in the dictionary. For instance, botanists classify most herbs as *"drugs."*

If you strictly go by the definition of the term, "drug," it is a substance or a medicine that has a physiological effect when introduced into the living body. Since it involves physiology or biological mechanisms, it relates to the manner by which a bodily part or a living organism functions. An example of which is the slowing down of your physiological reaction to anger or anxiety by making deep breaths.

With that said, we can now determine specifically the essential nature of Kratom.

1st thing you need to know...

First and foremost, Kratom is often mistaken as a drug. It is not! It is neither a synthetic substance nor a typical opiate. Instead, Kratom, per se, is an evergreen tropical plant—*"a naturally occurring plant medicine."*

2nd *thing you need to know...*

As a native plant growing predominantly in the Southeast Asian regions, it goes by its following respective ethnic names (refer to table below)

VERNACULAR	COMMON NAME
Filipino	Mambog
Vietnamese	Giam
Indonesian	Kadamba, Lugub, Puri
Malaysian	Kutum, Ketum, Polapupot, Biak-biak, Biak
Thai	Bai Karthom, Krataum, Taum, Kratom, Ketum, Ithang, Thang, Thom, Kakuan, Katuan

3rd *thing you need to know...*

Based on recorded history, Pieter Willem Korthals, a Dutch botanist, owns the credit for the official discovery of the Kratom plant. While working for the British East India Company, which exploited trade and commerce in the entire Oriental sphere, particularly in Southeast Asia, he described initially the Kratom plant in a publication curated by British naturalist Dr. George Darby Haviland in Sarawak, Malaysia in 1839.

In his description he highlighted that the natives of the region often used the Kratom plant as a traditional herbal medicine to relieve symptoms of diarrhea and as an effective pain relief. The plant is also known for enhancing physical endurance, libido, and extending duration of sexual intercourse.

Its common usage, however, became more popular for the treatment of opiate dependence, which was prevalent during those times. Patients consumed or chewed the Kratom leaves to produce a pleasant feeling, and thus, reduce their symptoms of withdrawals from opiate abuse.

Nowadays, processed Kratom is making waves into kava bars, festivals, and parties. Such socially vibrant places and events are where enthusiasts commonly use and/or abuse it to get a certain high.

4th thing you need to know...

Korthals classified Kratom in the same botanical family as coffee —Rubiaceae. He also designated the scientific name of Kratom as Mitragyna speciosa since it contains abundantly the opioid substance, mitragynine, which is the principal mood-altering compound in the plant.

5th thing you need to know...

The evergreen Kratom plant can grow to as tall as 80 feet (25m) and 15 feet (5m) wide. Its dark green and glossy leaves compose an average of a dozen to 17 pairs of veins.

6th thing you need to know...

The Kratom plant is indigenous to the Southeast Asian countries of Myanmar, Malaysia, and Thailand. It also thrives predominantly in Vietnam and Indonesia (particularly in Borneo, Bali, and its sovereign territories in New Guinea).

In the Philippines, its common sanctuaries are in the low-altitude forests in the main islands of Luzon, Visayas, and Mindanao. In the southwestern region of the Pacific Ocean, Kratom grows in some parts of Papua New Guinea, as well as in the outback locales of Australia and bush provinces of New Zealand.

7th thing you need to know...

The marketing of processed Kratom has not yet fully penetrated the global mainstream markets. Hence, its unregulated availability and commercial distribution usually end up in countless online shops. Kratom products can also be found in *head shops* (specialty stores selling paraphernalia used with illegal drugs).

Generally, they come in either tablet/pill or powder forms under various brands and packaged with health and vitality designs. Its business may be a new and flourishing industry, but authorities consider the commercial trading of Kratom as an underground economy due to current controversies of its legal use, which I will discuss later.

Chemical Characteristics & Core Compound Constituents

8th thing you need to know...

There are over 40 chemical compounds and at least 25 alkaloids in a Kratom leaf. Alkaloids are organic compounds that are generally basic or non-acidic (*i.e., cocaine, morphine, nicotine, and quinine*). Each of these compounds is renowned for their medicinal or poisonous attributes.

Of these alkaloids, *mitragynine* (66%), *speciogynine* (6.6%-7%), and *paynanthine* (8.6%-9%) are the most abundant. Studies showed that *mitragynine* is the key alkaloid directly responsible for much of the narcotic effects of Kratom. However, the two other components have vague properties as to how they exactly affect humans. Besides, both involve extreme complexities in a sustainable economic production.

9th thing you need to know...

Mitragynine and *7-hydroxymitragynine* are the chief psychoactive compounds in a Kratom leaf. On one hand, the quantities of *mitragynine* can vary greatly with the season of the year and the geographical location of growing and cultivating the plant.

Kratom plants originating from Southeast Asia tend to have higher amounts of *mitragynine*. If grown elsewhere, they generally have lower to non-existent *mitragynine* contents.

On the other hand, *7-hydroxymitragynine* only occurs in much lesser quantities in a Kratom leaf, with a measly amount of about 2% of its total alkaloids. Nonetheless, it acts as a reliable opioid competitor and characterizes to have the most potent analgesic effect.

10th *thing you need to know...*

Another noteworthy chemical compound in Kratom leaves is *epicatechin*. It is actually the same chemical constituent found in cranberry juice, green tea, and dark chocolate.

Epicatechin provides a broad range of health benefits — from decreasing the risks of cancer to reducing the detrimental influences of free radicals present in the body. Additionally, it is a very powerful antioxidant, which helps to prevent blockages in the arteries and oxidations of fat cells and tissues. It is also capable of impeding the growths of harmful microorganisms such as the E. coli bacteria.

Furthermore, *epicatechin* can help to resolve issues of urinary tract infections (UTIs). It can also be beneficial for people suffering from diabetes since it can resemble properties of insulin by biological mimicry. Equally significant is its vital role in inhibiting *alpha-amylase* (a saliva enzyme responsible for breaking down starches into sugars); and therefore, helps in the reduction of blood sugar levels.

Inherent Interactions

11th thing you need to know...

Both *mitragynine* and *7-hydroxymitragynine* compounds interact impulsively with the principal triumvirate of opioid receptors—*Mu, Delta, and Kappa*—in the human brain. Meaning to say, they cause certain effects similar to both stimulants and opioids. In particular, *mitragynine* acts as a stimulant while *7-hydroxymitragynine* acts as a sedative.

12th thing you need to know...

Therefore, these twin chemical compounds can ultimately produce a sense of euphoria, great pleasure and well-being, dreamlike states, reduced pain, and sedation. This is especially true when users consume larger dosages of Kratom.

13th thing you need to know...

Alternatively, when users take Kratom in smaller doses, they often report a heightened sense of sociability, increased energy, talkativeness, and alertness rather than sedation. Nonetheless, these essential Kratom contents can also result in uncomfortable, and sometimes, harmful side effects. Hence, the key lies in the proper administration of dosage.

Chapter 2: Specific Strains

There are currently several different strains of Kratom on the market. One reason for their overabundance is the practice of Kratom producers to combine two different types, and then, branding the resulting blends into new types with fancy names.

Another explanation could be the categorization of Kratom by its region of origin (*i.e., Red Indonesian, Green Sumatra, White Bali, etc.*).

14th thing you need to know...

Fact is that only three major specific strains compose the entire classification of Kratoms—White Vein, Green Vein, and Red Vein. Obviously, the details of the form and structure of a Kratom leaf determine and distinguish these principal strains from each other.

Clarifications in Colour Classification

Although it sounds logical to base the classification of Kratom strains from the specific color of its leaf veins, this does not always apply. Actually, it is more important to learn how each of these Kratom strains turns into their characteristic color.

15th thing you need to know...

The resulting strain color does not necessarily denote the original vein color. Kratom enthusiasts surmise that about 75% to 85% of the white and green strains available in the market are originally red-veined leaves.

A fine example is the Green Borneo. It is originally a red-veined leaf but dried in a specific process to attain its characteristic green color. Therefore, the original vein color is insignificant; what matters more is how farmers process the leaves after harvesting them.

16th thing you need to know...

Normally, growers dry greens inside an air-conditioned space with little to no lighting at all before drying them outside for an hour. Processing the whites usually involves drying the leaves indoors without lighting. Achieving the reds comes from either fermenting the leaves or subjecting them to various types and intensities of light exposure (*i.e., lamp light, sunlight or UV light*).

17*th thing you need to know...*

Other crucial factors in achieving specific strain colors are the source location of the plant, soil constitution, and season. Typically, the rainy seasons produce pale or brighter leaves, which are less potent. Conversely, harvested Kratoms during the dry seasons exhibit darker leaves that have narcotic effects and are more powerful.

While most of the white and green strains originated from red-veined leaves, there actually exist white- and green-veined leaves. These leaf species are just usually rare to find.

In conclusion, the drying process of farming Kratom leaves is the key to changing the colors of the strains. Growers will only have white, green, red, and *Bentuangie* (fermented red-veined leaf).

Watery Whites

18*th thing you need to know...*

White Vein Kratom (Tang Gua): White Kratom is in the opposite side of red Kratom in the Kratom strain spectrum. It denotes having sufficient water volumes during its entire life cycle; thus, it has low *7-hydroxymitragynine* levels. For this reason, producers usually blend it with a green or red strain to attain potent effects of the scanty alkaloid.

Provided Potencies:
- Acts as a mild caffeine substitute
- Causes muscle relaxation
- Improves mental focus and attention spans
- Increases alertness, wakefulness, and creativity
- Battles social fretfulness and builds confidence
- Relieves pain and irritating feelings
- Enhances overall mood with euphoric effects

Preferred Practitioners/Patients:
- Heavy users of caffeine
- Sufferers of opioid withdrawals
- Individuals experiencing pain symptoms
- People undergoing stress/depression and anxiety

Generous Greens

19th thing you need to know...

Green Vein Kratom (Yakyai): Noted as the middle of the road strain between the white and red Kratoms, it is neither an option that is the least nor the most expensive. In brief, it is a moderate strain. It is popular for its more sophisticated flavor compared to the slightly bitter taste of red Kratom.

Green Kratom has more balanced potent effects since it contains generously equal levels of alkaloids. As such, blending green Kratoms is ideal for achieving the full effects of each combined leaf. Typically, green Kratom is a blend of both red and white Kratoms.

Provided Potencies:
- Possesses similar applications as white Kratoms, but with more intense effects

Preferred Practitioners/Patients:
- Recommended to the same white Kratom users, but with a more pleasurable experience

Regional Reds

20th *thing you need to know...*

Red Vein Kratom (Kan Daeng): Red Kratom is specifically regional, solely a Thai produce. It is the most popular and best-selling Kratom strain. Its distinctive characteristic is its ability to grow in any environmental types, be it in water or dry areas.

Essentially, red Kratoms are sedatives. Its natural effect of numbing—similar to that of morphine—to relieve pain symptoms heightens more its repute as a potent sedative rather than a stimulant.

Provided Potencies:
- Possesses the most potent effects attributed by both white and green Kratoms, except that it is a powerful sedative, albeit, effects of milder mood enhancements also arise from the strain.

Preferred Practitioners/Patients:
- Highly advisable for opiate-dependent patients since it matches most of the sensory effects of opiate with only lesser side effects

Stimulating Strains

21st thing you need to know...

Maeng Da and Thai Kratoms: Maeng Da Kratom is a genetically enhanced type of Thai Kratom. Commercially, the red and green Maeng

Da Kratoms are blends containing a white strain.

Scientific evaluations reveal that the addition of the white strain makes Maeng Da the most potent stimulating strain of Kratoms. It is also ideal as a mood enhancer and pain reliever while acting as an excellent strain for revitalizing the user.

Thai Kratom is a powerful energy booster. Like Maeng Da, it has intense pain-killing properties. The white/green blend Thai Kratom is also a powerful stimulant for countering anxiety and depression. However, it is deficient with analgesic qualities.

Sedating Strains

22nd thing you need to know...

Indo, Bali and Borneo Kratoms: Borneo Kratom is a stronger muscle relaxant than an Indo Kratom. It also has its own distinctive odor, which is easy to recognize. It is a versatile sedating strain, serving as a pain reliever and mood enhancer with lesser side effects.

The Bali Kratom is the most economical, mainly because of its rapid growth and larger leaf size qualities. Administering its proper dosage can be tricky since it has a very low threshold to effect wobbling. As a resolve, experts usually counter the downside by combining it with other strains.

Chapter 3: Prescriptive Preparations & Ideal Ingestions

The market offers two principal processed forms of Kratom —powder, and extract—aside from the native leaf itself. Users take these common formulations in the following manners:

Leaf of Life

23rd thing you need to know...

Fresh or Dried Leaves: You can either smoke or chew a fresh or dried Kratom leaf.

Smoking – In order to smoke Kratom, you need to crush a dried Kratom leaf and roll the particles with another dried leaf. However, this method is impractical due to the substantive and unregulated dosages of the leaves that you can smoke easily.

Chewing – Users can cut out the fibrous and stringy central vein of a freshly picked Kratom leaf before chewing it. After juicing it from chewing, you can swallow the chewed material and follow it up by drinking coffee, tea, or water.

Typically, you may chew one to three fresh leaves for acquiring effects of vigor and euphoria. However, since dried Kratom leaves have rough texture, you may prefer to crush them up first into powder to facilitate the ease of swallowing.

Power Powder

24th thing you need to know...

Powdered Form: You can make powdered Kratom easily by putting dried Kratom—either whole or crushed or coarsely ground leaves—in your coffee grinder or kitchen blender. Thereafter, process the leaves for about 5 minutes or more at high speed.

Prepared for the Toss-N'-Wash Method – This is the quickest, simplest, and easiest way to consume Kratom. It is also the best method to attain the effects faster.

You only have to measure your desired or recommended dose and pour it into your mouth. Swallow it up immediately with a swig of water.

Alternatively, you may prefer dividing your dose into two mouthfuls rather than doing it in a single go. The lesser Kratom powder you pour in your mouth, the easier for you to take a swig and swallow.

Prepared as Tablet/Capsule or Pill – Several suppliers offer powdered Kratom leaves in the forms of tablets or pills. They also sell plain, finely powdered Kratom. You can put refined Kratom into capsules. This is your ideally convenient method for avoiding the taste of Kratom, this also works best for people on the go.

However, the drawback to using this formulation is the various sizes and capacities of capsules. For instance, a size-00 capsule only contains 0.5 grams of powder. Hence, if your recommended dosage would be 5 grams, then you need to consume 10 capsules to attain the desired effect.

25th thing you need to know...

Kratom Powder Blended with Water or Other Beverages: Among the most common practices for this formulation are the following:

Prepared as Paste — Here is a recipe to prepare powdered Kratom paste for drinking:

1. In a small empty drinking glass, place a single dose of powdered Kratom.

2. Pour just enough water to create a soft paste. Stir the mixture to let the powder absorb the water completely or until achieving a homogenized paste consistency.

3. By using a spoon, scoop an easy-to-swallow paste into your mouth. Take immediately a big swig with a glass of water.

4. Repeat scooping, swigging, and swallowing until you have consumed the entire dose.

NOTE: Be careful not to take too much scooped paste all at once to avoid choking accidentally on the mixture.

Prepared as Slurry/Smoothie — Here is recipe to prepare powdered Kratom as slurry or smoothie:

1. Add your typical dose of powdered

Kratom to a glass filled with 8 ounces of water or other beverage.

2. Stir thoroughly until the powder is completely suspended. Take a quick swig before it has a chance to settle.

3. Add ½-cup of water to the glass to wash and recover any particles sticking to the sides. Stir and drink.

4. Chase away the bitter taste by sipping a fruit juice or chewing a mint-flavored gum.

Prepared as Protein Shake – Although most users claim to enjoy better effects ingesting Kratom mixed with protein shakes, the blend actually has more calories. Just the same, this formulation, especially made with chocolate milk, is the most pleasant and tastiest way to ingest Kratom.

Chocolate milk masks remarkably well Kratom's bitter taste. Besides, its viscosity is ideal in helping to prevent the Kratom from settling, even when stirring the mixture. However, to create a smooth milkshake without the lumps of powdered Kratom floating on top, follow this simple procedure:

1. Put a dose of powdered Kratom into an empty glass. Pour an equal volume of chocolate milk in the glass. (Typically, use 1-cup [8-fl. oz.] of chocolate milk per dose of Kratom.)

2. Stir thoroughly until the powdered Kratom absorbs the liquid completely or until achieving a homogenized paste consistency.

3. Add more tablespoons of chocolate milk. Stir again to a smooth consistency free of lumps.

4. Pour the rest of the chocolate milk. Stir again until thoroughly mixed. Drink until the glass is empty. (You can add a little chocolate milk to the glass to wash and recover any particles sticking to the sides. Stir and drink.)

NOTE: Non-dairy, chocolate-flavored almond milk is also a better alternative for chocolate milk.

Prepared as Juice – Kratom powder or extract

can blend well with fresh juice. You can mix it up with your favorite fruits and choice of a couple of vegetables. You only need your reliable kitchen blender and you are already good to go.

For starters, take inspiration from this simple Kratom fruit and vegetable juice recipe:

Combine all the following ingredients into a blender, and process the mixture for about a minute or until thoroughly blended:

1. Kratom powder

2. One apple, roughly chopped
3. 2 carrots, roughly chopped

4. Juice of one lemon

5. A handful of kale or spinach, roughly chopped

6. Pinch of ginger powder

NOTE: You can also mix powdered Kratom with applesauce, milk, yogurt, and *kefir* (a creamy drink made of fermented cow's milk, or sometimes, goat's milk).

Tea Treat

26th thing you need to know...

Kratom Tea: You can also brew or infuse dried Kratom leaves with hot or cold water and drink it as tea. Historically, the practice of concocting an effective Kratom tea involves combining a dose of Kratom with 8 to 10 ounces of water and allowing it to steep for about 10 minutes at high-simmer or 15 minutes at a low boil, and then straining the leaves to produce the tea.

However, I suggest making Kratom Tea using this recipe:

1. Put 2 ounces (56 grams) of dried, crushed or coarsely ground Kratom leaves into a pot. Pour 1 a liter of water and boil the mixture for about 15 minutes.

2. Pour the tea through a strainer into a bowl. Squeeze the leaves in the strainer to drain most of the liquid out. Reserve the liquid.

3. Put the strained leaves back in the pot. Pour another liter of fresh water and boil again for 15 minutes.

4. Repeat Step-2. Discard the leaves. Combine both reserved liquids by pouring them back into the pot. Boil until reducing the volume to about 1 cup (250 mL).

NOTE: The technique of boiling down to a small volume is to allow swallowing each individual dose quickly. This recipe produces enough tea for about eight moderately strong doses, if using Kratom leaves of 'premium quality'.

However, you can boil the tea down to your desired concentration. Just be careful when nearing the end of the boiling process. When the tea begins to be syrupy, it may spatter and/or burn. You can also apply this general preparation method with larger or smaller amounts of Kratom; simply adjust the volume of water used.

Kratom tea tastes bitter, so you can sweeten it by adding honey or sugar. However, if you prefer, you can drink it quickly with one gulp and chase it quickly with your choice of drink.

You can store Kratom tea safely in the refrigerator for about a week or more. You can even store it for several months, for as long as you add about 10% alcohol to preserve it. That is adding one part of 80-proof liquor (*i.e., rum or vodka*) to three parts of Kratom tea.

When refrigerating Kratom tea, some of its components may settle at the bottom of the container. The sediments formed actually contain active Kratom alkaloids so you should dissolve it again before drinking by warming it up and stirring it.

Exhilarating Extract

27th thing you need to know...

Kratom Syrup or Resin Extract: You can prepare syrup for preparing Kratom tea. You only need to boil the tea further and obtain its syrupy substance.

You can always store this syrup in your refrigerator for later use. The common usage of Kratom syrup is for smoking it in a pipe, similar to the procedure of smoking opium.

If you would evaporate the water from the Kratom Tea completely, you will achieve small pellets of resin-like extracts. This can later be prepared as a liquid dose or as a sweetened Kratom ball. Some people chose to swallow the pellet directly or dissolve it in hot water, and drink it as tea.

28th *thing you need to know...*

Kratom Food Recipe Mix: The taste of the Kratom extract and powder can be quite challenging to your taste buds. You can use Kratom in certain food recipes. One of my favorites is the Oatmeal Kratom. Follow the recipe below for preparation:

1. Put 5 to 7 grams of Kratom powder in a bowl. Add a cup of dry or instant oats.

2. Pour heated water or milk into the mixture. Stir thoroughly for 3 to 5 minutes or until fully cooking the oatmeal.

3. Add honey, brown sugar, or stevia extract to sweeten. For an enhanced texture, add some nuts or blueberries.

Chapter 4: Pharmacological Properties

The extensive medicinal properties of Kratom are still continuously undergoing further studies and development.

However, what we can be certain of, as described in Chapter 2, is that Kratom has evolved into wider varieties of strains due to its varying farming processes or breeding techniques, as well as its geographical growth origins.

As a result, each of these strains can broadly differ in its pharmacological effects —categorized principally into moderate, sedating, and stimulating.

29th *thing you need to know...*

Similar to all psychoactive agents, differing dosages can produce a range of effects. The moderate use of Kratom appears to neither promote violent tendencies nor impair motor control. Small dosages of Kratom create feelings of alertness and mild stimulation, while larger doses result in sedated feelings.

Strong Sensory Stimulant & Soothing Sedative States

30th thing you need to know...

According to Kratom connoisseurs, red Kratoms are more sedating; whereas, green and white Kratoms are the more stimulating strains.

31st thing you need to know...

Stimulant State: At this dosage level, Kratom differs from other stimulants of the central nervous system (CNS) like amphetamine drugs, caffeine, and cocoa. It is more inclined to influence the cognitive rather than physical aspects, as follows:

- Heightens alertness and consciousness
- Boosts physical, as well as sexual energies
- Motivates the will to get things done
- Improves abilities of monotonous performances
- Raises positive mood levels
- Staves off stress, depression, and anxiety
- Increases confidence and sociability levels

32nd *thing you need to know...*

Sedative State: At this dosage level, Kratom induces your body to feel euphoric states while enhances its analgesic qualities:

- Reduces sensitivity to emotional or physical pain
- Triggers dispositions of tranquility and relaxation
- Induces overall feelings of comfort and pleasure
- Introduces an enjoyable daydream like state
- Enhances the appreciation levels for music

This dosage can also have side effects, which include:

- Profuse sweating or itching
- Smaller or constricted eye pupils
- Nauseated feelings, but it could subside quickly when you lie down and relax

Definitive Doses

33rd *thing you need to know...*

The appropriate quantities of Kratom that you should be purchasing must be in accordance with the frequency of your intended usage. However, it is highly advisable not to use Kratom daily.

At the earliest instance, it is always better to stay on the side of caution than to commit mistakes or take the risks with incorrect dosage, especially if you are a beginner.

Image below will show you a general guide of the potency comparisons of the most common Kratom strains available in the market:

Kratom Strain	Energy Potency, %	Sedative Potency, %	Pain Relief Potency, %
Red Maeng Da	20	75	90
Red Sumatra	30	70	75
Red Indonesian	35	60	65
Red Vein Thai	50	45	55
Green Horned Leaf	85	5	50
Green Maeng Da	90	10	60
Green Sumatra	65	30	50
Green Indonesian	60	40	35
Green Vein Thai	60	35	35
White Horned Leaf	85	20	20
White Maeng Da	40	75	45
White Sumatra	65	40	45
White Bali	65	25	30
White Vein Thai	70	30	30

34th thing you need to know...

A safe usage guideline would be using Kratom not more than once or twice per week. Much preferably, never take it more than once or twice in a month, but I suggest you seek a professional opinion of a doctor or a medical professional before ingesting or self-prescribing.

The side effects of ingesting Kratom too often can lead you to develop strong dependencies on Kratom. Moreover, you would only be inclined to swap out effectively one addiction for another, especially if you use Kratom in averting withdrawal symptoms from narcotics such as heroin.

In short, reserve using Kratom as a special, yet, occasional treat. Infrequent usage of Kratom will assure you to receive more pleasure while avoiding addiction or the development of an increased tolerance.

35th thing you need to know...

For your proper guidance, refer to Tables-3 and 4 for the recommended oral dosages typical of the current Kratom varieties.

Table 3

STRAIN	EFFECT	DOSAGE
Bali	Euphoric, most classic opiate-like	½ - 3 teaspoons
Maeng Da	Energizing, stimulating, pain-killing	½ - 3 teaspoons
Red Vein Thai	Similar to Bali	½ - 3 teaspoons
Red Vein Bali	Sedating, opiate-like	½ - 3 teaspoons
Green Vein Bali	Stimulating, pain-killing	½ - 3 teaspoons
White Vein Bali	More euphoric	½ - 3 teaspoons
White Vein Thai	Euphoric, stimulating	½ - 3 teaspoons
Super Indo	Similar to Bali, but less euphoric	½ - 3 teaspoons
Super Green Malaysian	Stimulating and less euphoric	½ - 3 teaspoons
Ultra-Enhanced Indo	Most euphoric and reduces social anxiety	1g or less if mixed with powdered leaf

Ultra-Enhanced Maeng Da	Powerfully stimulating and pain-killing	1g or less if mixed with powdered leaf
Thai Essence	Similar to Maeng Da kick	1g or less if mixed with powdered leaf
Full Spectrum Tincture (FST)	Ulta-Enhanced Undo in liquid form	0.25ml or more

Table 4

PREMIUM QUALITY KRATOM	
INTENSITY OF EFFECTS	DOSAGE
Threshold	2-4 gm
Mild	3-5 gm
Moderate	4-10 gm
Strong	8-15 gm
Very Strong	12-25 gm
ULTRA POTENT KRATOM	
INTENSITY OF EFFECTS	DOSAGE
Threshold	1-3 gm
Mild	2-4 gm
Moderate	3-7 gm
Strong	6-10 gm
Very Strong	8-16 gm
KRATOM EXTRACT	
INTENSITY OF EFFECTS	DOSAGE
Threshold	1 gm
Mild	1-2 gm
Moderate	2-4 gm
Strong	3-6 gm
Very Strong	5-8 gm

36th *thing you need to know...*

To distinguish the classified intensity of effects please consider:

- **Threshold** – denotes apparent, yet, subtle effects
- **Mild** – implies typically stimulant-like effects
- **Moderate** – connotes effects can be either sedative-euphoric-analgesic or stimulant-like
- **Strong** – describes sedative | euphoric | analgesic effects; intensively strong for highly sensitive users
- **Very Strong** – signifies powerful sedative | euphoric | analgesic effects; intensively strong for most users

Satisfy Sensitivities & Thwart Tolerances: Proper Practices

37th *thing you need to know...*

Sensitivity and tolerance to Kratom will vary for each individual user. If you are hypersensitive to Kratom, then you may experience certain adverse reactions like vomiting or an upset stomach.

38th *thing you need to know...*

As recommended, you should always begin your Kratom intake with a low dose. You should also take the same advice when you are sampling with a new batch or set of Kratom.

39th *thing you need to know...*

When consuming high doses of Kratom, it is ideal to take it on an empty stomach or about 3 hours after eating. Alternatively, take it in the morning or around a couple of hours before eating.

Although you can take it with food, it results in reduced effects. In this case, your body tends to develop a tolerance that requires taking higher doses than normal to attain the desired effect.

40th *thing you need to know...*

Regardless of which powdered Kratom you buy, never chase the high, and most importantly always talk to a medical practitioner before taking any medications.

41st *thing you need to know...*

As a general dosage guide, especially for new Kratom users, the crucial thing is to find out your recommended dose for a particular Kratom strain. The following procedures will help you discover your required Kratom dosage if you are going to self-medicate:

Step-1: On an empty stomach, take about 2-3 grams of Kratom powder. After 20 to 30 minutes, you will notice its effects (This step is mandatory every time you try taking a new Kratom strain.)

Step-2: Evaluate these effects or sensations after about 45 minutes to an hour. If you feel nothing, then increase the dosage; add about 1 to 2 grams.

Step-3: Reevaluate the effects after 15 minutes. If you deem it necessary to increase a bit of the dosage, then add about 0.5 to 2 grams.

Step-4: At this stage, you should already feel something more pleasurable! Yet, after about 4 to 5 hours, you might want to take more. Repeat Step-3 and add a little more, using the same Kratom strain, but please be very careful not to overdose, especially if you are new to trying Kratom.

42nd thing you need to know...

As a rule of thumb, especially for beginners, 3 to

5 grams of Kratom powder is enough as an introductory dosage for your brain's fresh receptors. If you weigh less than 150 lbs., then 1.5 grams will be your sufficient dosage to start out.

43rd thing you need to know...

When using Kratom irregularly, or for those who tend to rotate their consumption for different strains, the same safe dosage of 1.5 grams is advisable to start with each strain.

Tolerance, however, is temporary. A few days or weeks of abstinence can resume to normal sensitivity levels. Just the same, you ought to avoid any tolerances to Kratom before they defeat your purpose.

With that said, it is important to learn how to use Kratom efficiently and effectively without succumbing to any forms of tolerances. Aside from determining your dosage quantities, as discussed earlier, you should consider spacing and rotating your dosage to prevent acquiring a heavy tolerance.

44th thing you need to know...

Kratom Dosage Spacing: Spacing out your

dosage ensures your brain receptors keep on performing with their baseline/normal reaction levels. Thus, you will have no tendencies of increasing your tolerance. Regardless of treatment issues, it is wiser to restrict Kratom use to only once per day if you have been a "heavy user." Taking it twice a month at the most would be preferable for new users.

45th thing you need to know...

Kratom Strain Rotation: Some "heavy users" found success in preventing tolerance by altering strains used each time. This ensures to vary the behaviors or reaction levels of brain receptors. As such, the brain treats each subjected strain as a new element to process.

For instance, avoid using permanently a single strain, say, a Red vein Thai; instead, switch to a Green vein Bali as an alternate for your subsequent use. Ideally, you need to have at least four varieties of strains to use in rotating order.

Aside from stopping to build tolerance, strain rotation reduces the possibilities of experiencing *'strain-burnout.'* This is a detrimental condition where you become almost immune to any of the effects of a specific Kratom strain.

Efficacious Effectivity

46th thing you need to know...

Whenever you ingest any variety of Kratom, it typically takes you from 20 to 40 minutes to experience the onrush of any sensations related to what you have consumed. As soon as you sense these feelings, the effects will last for between 3 to 6 hours.

47th thing you need to know...

When taking Kratom on an empty stomach, you will feel the onset of the effects 30 to 40 minutes after ingestion. When ingesting Kratom on a full stomach, effects usually begin 60-90 minutes after ingestion.

48th thing you need to know...

When taken in either gelatin or vegetarian capsules, the effects are much delayed than usual since it takes more time for the capsules to dissolve in your stomach.

49th thing you need to know...

In general, effects of white Kratom last for about

3 hours; red Kratom for roughly 5 hours; and, green Kratom can last for as long as 8 hours.

50th thing you need to know...

However, effectivity of the Kratom ingested depends on how accustomed you are to the effects of each Kratom strain. If you have developed tolerances to the different strains, you will most likely feel much less of an impact than you would have when first taking the supplement.

Current Costs

51st thing you need to know...

A crucial point to note in the pricing of Kratom depends on quantity, quality, and the type of Kratom. Foremost, the prices of Kratom capsules are much different from plain powder, extracts, leaves, resins, or tinctures. Although loose powders and the contents of the capsule are almost similar, capsules are costlier since you can take them conveniently in pill form.

52nd thing you need to know...

The prevailing price of Kratom powder ranges

from $12 to $21 per ounce.

Capsulated Kratoms cost an average of $16 per 1-ounce bottle.

Kratom resins cost around $15 per 15 grams (this means it takes 15 grams of Kratom leaves to make pure Kratom resin).

Kratom tinctures or concentrates go for as low as $100 per 6ml bottle to as high as $430 per 30ml bottle.

Kratom extracts are more expensive than the classical Kratom powder because they are super-concentrated preparations. The upside to taking it is in smaller doses to attain desired effects. Generally, the full dose ranges between 0.5 gm and 1 gram. Meaning, its ultimate price turns out the same as those powders per dose.

53rd thing you need to know...

In comparison to most medical drugs, Kratom is much less expensive. This price advantage derives from the fact that you only need to take smaller doses of Kratom to feel the effects instantly. Unlike other medical drugs, your doctor addresses your health issue with several medicines for you to buy and take them within a definite duration, which often stretches for weeks. In the end, these prescribed medical drugs can really hurt your pocket!

54th thing you need to know...

Therefore, when you look for Kratom products at their best prices and receive the ultimate value for your money, common sense dictates that you ought to compare the price with the quality of the product. In addition, since the marketing of Kratom exists predominantly in online shops, you should know the reliability and trustworthiness of these sources.

Finding ways to buy and use Kratom effectively can be challenging. It involves lots of trial and error; so, when purchasing Kratom, please ensure to do your due diligence on the trustworthiness of the company/website where you will be purchasing.

Chapter 5: Bonuses & Benefits

Kratoms recent appearance on the news has attracted a lot of attention. A recent publication by CNN has detailed the beneficial impacts Kratoms have had on the lives of a multitude of people worldwide suffering from debilitating pain and those struggling with narcotics addiction, particularly opium, heroin, and amphetamine abuses. This caused quite a stir and started a debate as to the benefits and dangers of using Kratom. Let's explore those now.

Inflammatory Illnesses Inhibitor

55th *thing you need to know...*

Kratom has a diversity of medicinal effects due to its unique profile of organic compounds. As a versatile herbal medicine, it serves as a strong agent for inhibiting a variety of illnesses largely attributed to inflammation:

- Anticonvulsant (relaxes the muscles)
- Antidepressant (alleviates depression)
- Antidiarrheal (treats diarrhea)
- Anti-inflammatory (reduces inflammation)
- Antileukemic (acts against leukemia)
- Antimalarial (prevents malaria)
- Antipyretic (relieves fever)
- Antitussive (suppresses a cough)
- Anxiolytic (reduces anxiety)
- Boosts energy levels
- Lifts up moods to euphoric heights
- Stimulates immune system
- Lowers hypertension and blood sugar levels
- Nootropic (enhances cognitive functions)
- Opiate maintenance (as a substitute substance)
- Opiate withdrawal relief
- Pain relief

Traditional Therapies & Treatments

56th *thing you need to know...*

Historically, early users of Kratom found its leaves as effective treatments to overcome stress. In particular, male manual laborers used Kratom to enhance their physical endurance as a means of averting the stresses of hard work.

57th thing you need to know...

Early wellness documents in Malaysia and Thailand also reveal that the application of Kratom has become an affordable and popular alternative substance for using opium. Nevertheless, there have never been any substantive clinical tests and medical studies to help people understand the extensive health effects of Kratom.

Even the future expectations of Kratom assessed by both the U.S. Food and Drug Administration (FDA) and the Drug Enforcement Administration (DEA) appear to be gloomy. Yet, there has been a slew of recorded benefits for using or taking Kratom in specific forms. Some of the principal applications include:

58th thing you need to know...

Therapy for Opiate Addiction: Kratom has been increasingly popular among people suffering from opiate addiction and trying to get off the hook of illegal drugs. The compounds in the Kratom leaf help to reduce the side effects of opium withdrawal as they mimic most of the sensations and effects that opioids provide to users.

In Asia, many recovering drug addicts chew Kratom leaves that produce a consistent and psychological effect to battle the symptoms of opiate withdrawal. Additionally, compared to using harsher drugs, the method of chewing the leaves provides a safe and instant boost related to their addiction.

59th thing you need to know...

In comparison to opioid use, *respiratory depression* or slowed breathing has never been part of the effects of Kratom use. Respiratory depression is a typical and deadly factor in opioids abuse since opium has the ability to shut down the respiratory system, particularly during an overdose.

60th thing you need to know...

As confirmed by research, Kratom can have addictive qualities, only because of its pleasurable effects. Sometimes, this type of addiction is simply an interpretation of a developing tolerance for heavy and daily users. Fact is that nearly none of the plant's elements is addictive. Thus, in reality, the abuse potential of Kratom can be very low.

61ˢᵗ *thing you need to know...*

Since Kratom is an unregulated product, only a few studies about the plant are reliable. However, many anecdotal reports support the beneficial role of Kratom in helping people to overcome opioid withdrawals.

62ⁿᵈ *thing you need to know...*

The American Association of Pharmaceutical Scientists (AAPS) confirmed that alkaloid compounds in Kratom could bond easily to opioid receptors in the body. As such, these compounds cause the release of *dopamine* and *serotonin* (chemical substances responsible for transmitting nerve impulses in certain brain cells to help control moods and emotions, as well as to regulate movement), just as opioid drugs typically do.

Kratom however releases the substance at more manageable levels compared to heroin or prescription pills. Thus, the symptoms of opium withdrawal become less severe.

63ʳᵈ *thing you need to know...*

Acute and Chronic Pain Reliever: The most important and popular reason for using Kratom is the effectiveness of its opium-like qualities for alleviating pain. Pharmaceutical studies actually concluded favorable evaluations for using the rich analgesic properties of Kratom leaves in the self-treatment of chronic pains typically experienced in abrupt withdrawals of opioid abuse.

64*th* thing you need to know...

Kratom leaves quickly relieve pain throughout a person's body by influencing the systemic activities of hormones. When chewing the leaves, the quantities of *dopamine* and *serotonin* compounds released increases. Essentially, the Kratom alkaloids act in a morphine-like way by dulling the pain receptors all over the body.

65*th* thing you need to know...

Energy Booster: The Kratom leaf compounds virtually heighten focus and a buzzing stimulation that increase productivity levels. These inherent sensations of an energy boost experienced through using Kratom are entirely different from other stimulating substances. Kratom aficionados termed it singularly as, "Kratom high."

66*th* thing you need to know...

Unlike a caffeine overdose or simply consuming too much caffeine, Kratom does not tend to increase the heart rate. Such a unique quality arises from the extract's metabolic processes, which calm the nerves while increasing oxygen supply in the bloodstream for a more stable energy boost.

67th thing you need to know...

Enhances the Mood and Relieves Anxiety: For the same reason that the properties of the compounds in the plant help to boost energy and relieve pain, Kratom also helps people suffering from severe nervousness or anxiety, depression, and mood swings. The compounds in Kratom actually target to affect the brain's neurotransmitters—nerves that transmit signals for regulating emotions.

In particular, the leaf extracts augment the release of hormones throughout the body to control mood swings in more restrained ways, if not, eliminating them.

68th thing you need to know...

With each strain producing different effects, a new and inexperienced user may choose the wrong strain to treat their desired symptoms.

For your quick guide in relieving anxiety, your best bet includes the Bali, Indo, and some varieties of red vein Kratoms. Please refer back to Image-3.

69th *thing you need to know...*

Sexual Activity Enhancer: Traditionally, Kratom practitioners have long branded the wonder plant as an aphrodisiac. Its botanical properties were renowned to aid in premature ejaculation, as well as increasing fertility in men.

While there have been no scientific studies showing evidence of its sexual effects, laboratory studies on animals revealed an increased production of sperm cells. Besides, the market for using Kratom for sexual enhancements has been growing steadily over the years. This market growth apparently manifests and strengthens its repute as an effective aphrodisiac.

Chapter 6: Prudent & Precautionary Practices

Recently, Kratom has also gained popularity among the younger generations for its euphoric effects that provide a 'legal' high. Its status as an alternative to other stimulant and sedative type of drugs is also of equal interest.

Misuse Measures

70th thing you need to know...

Merchants sell Kratom products in a wide variety of forms. As a result, Kratom products can often vary in their respective alkaloid concentrations. Thus, always be aware and beware of certain misleading product labels and the marketing hypes. Some vendors sell bogus products by adulterating Kratom with other chemicals or herbs or misrepresenting other herbs as Kratom.

71st thing you need to know...

Chemical analysis on some Kratom products has revealed many forms of adulterations with other substances. In most cases, suppliers remove certain amounts of the original Kratom contents and replace them with less expensive herbs or other similar substance to cut down retailers' costs and increase profits.

72nd *thing you need to know…*

In other cases, suppliers add synthetic or designer drugs to enhance the effects further. These, deceptive products, misleadingly labeled as 'pure Kratom extracts' actually contain the synthetic drug, *O-desmethyltramadol*—a fatally potent synthetic opioid. One concoction goes by the label, *'Krypton,'* which compose Kratom leaves mixed with the drug.

73rd *thing you need to know…*

Disturbingly, products containing this drug have resulted in a long list of recorded deaths (with the first fatality accounted in Sweden). Yet, Kratom in its original form is far from dangerous and there has been no single reported case resulting in death after its use.

74th *thing you need to know…*

Other studies have also found similar deadly compounds—specifically morphine and *hydrocodone* (a semi-synthetic drug sourced from opium derivatives)—laced in other Kratom products. Since these are prime constituents of opioid compounds, their effects are somehow akin to those of Kratom.

75th thing you need to know...

While Kratom is a relatively safe and tremendously useful herb, it is just unfortunate that some unscrupulous merchants and reckless suppliers are acting so irresponsibly. If you are thinking of purchasing Kratom products, ensure to purchase from traders or shops that conduct routine testing prior to retailing the products sourced from suppliers.

Critical Concerns & Conditions

Clinical studies are significant for the development and promotion of new drugs. They help to determine consistently the harmful effects and interactions with other drugs. These studies also help to recognize effective dosages that are sustainable and less dangerous.

Studies have found that alkaloids induce physical

effects on humans. Kratom contains nearly as many alkaloids as hallucinogenic mushrooms and opium. Thus, it bears the powerful ability to have a potent effect on the human body.

Although some of these effects are desirable, others may be causes for great concern. This gives rise to why the necessity for extensive and further studies on Kratom is indeed urgent.

76th thing you need to know...

However, there have never been any in-depth studies about Kratom. Hence, there are no recorded official recommendations for its medical use up to now. Instead, the truth of the matter is that the limited information on the benefits and risks of Kratom in humans run counter to the over-sensationalized and inaccurate reports by popular media about the intricacies of Kratom use.

77th thing you need to know...

Due to the lack of sufficient evidence and available confirmations of its safe usage, it then becomes a careful forethought to keep Kratom off the reach of children. The same precautionary measures would be advisable for women undergoing pregnancy or lactation. For, after all, it is unknown whether Kratom could cause fetal death or birth defects.

Safeness & Sustainability

78*th* *thing you need to know...*

If you consume Kratom by itself, which is without any combination of other drugs, then your only greatest risk is falling asleep without warning. The perceived problems arise when you engage in hazardous activities while under a slight or heavy influence of Kratom. Therefore, you should use your common sense and refrain from driving a vehicle, using power tools, scaling ladders, or leaving a pot/kettle on a lit stove, operating heavy machinery, and all things alike.

79*th* *thing you need to know...*

Health issues are least likely to occur in occasional users of Kratom unless, of course, users consume large quantities of Kratom daily. Like any other medicine, reactions vary in each individual. Some people might have unusual reactions to Kratom or an allergy despite using it responsibly.

Those who are heavily dependent on it will

eventually develop dark facial pigmentations and an unhealthy weight loss. Worse, they incur physical withdrawal symptoms when quitting the habit abruptly. These withdrawal symptoms may include crying, diarrhea, muscle aches and jerking, irritability, and a runny nose.

Toxicological Truths

Similar to its safe medical use, scientific research on the toxicity and adverse effects of Kratom are still also limited. We can only contend with consuming a few of the facts surfacing from trusted publications and medical reports.

80th thing you need to know...

Primarily, a 2015 literary review from the International Journal of Legal Medicine considered that Kratom is minimally toxic. It concluded that the pharmacological effects of the Kratom leaves are dose-dependent. Meaning, the more a user takes them, the stronger the effect will be.

Although there were some reported cases of deaths attributed to heavy Kratom use, there was neither solid proof nor accounts provided where Kratom solely contributed to the fatalities. A study in Thailand, however, documented cases of adverse withdrawal symptoms and Kratom poisoning among its users.

81st thing you need to know...

Most of the complaints of withdrawal symptoms and Kratom poisoning were under the influence of other prescribed substances or illicit drugs like codeine or cough syrup. During the last decade, there were nine death cases of intoxication related to the use of the deadly Kratom-based product, *Krypton*. However, the reports ascribed these fatalities to the addition of a synthetic opioid, which is the usual element blended in the product.

Strength Sports

82nd thing you need to know...

Kratom's reach also extends to professional sports. The plant's analgesic and stimulating effects only imply that Kratom can be beneficial for enhancing performances in certain sports disciplines.

Technically, it is possible to detect Kratom alkaloids in body fluids. For the first time, in

2015, sports officials chanced upon detecting the essential element of Kratom—*mitragynine*—in four doping control samples coming from strength sports, particularly powerlifting and weightlifting.

However, since most places legalize Kratom as an herbal drug, it need not undergo normal testing. Protocols may likely change, especially when Kratom eventually becomes a regulated substance in the U. S.

Chapter 7: Aftereffects Assessments

Considering all the positive effects occurring in Kratom use, it is important that we also highlight its negative effects.

One of the side effects of using Kratom is the notorious *'Kratom hangover,'* which carries similar symptoms typical to an alcoholic hangover. The following are the common assessments of the top five aftereffects of Kratom use:

Chronic Consumers' Conditions

83rd *thing you need to know...*

High-dosage users generally experience irritability and anxiety due to Kratom's stimulating effects. Long-term users usually incur anorexia and abnormal weight loss, facial hyperpigmentation, and fretting, trembling, or wobbling.

Furthermore, the reported negative side effects extend to include alternating chills and sweats, constipation, dehydration, dizziness, itching, mouth and throat numbness, nausea, sedation, stomachaches, tiredness, unsteadiness, visual alterations and vomiting. For regular users, some have become vulnerable to develop tolerance, and very often, they inevitably increase their usual dosages over time. Others simply succumb to addiction.

Addictive Aspects

In recent years, the use of Kratom expanded from Asia towards the U.S. and Europe. Since then, there have been steadily increasing reports of users becoming addicted or physically dependent on Kratom.

84th thing you need to know...

The main culprit for this possible addiction is the opioid-like analgesic effects of Kratom. Even though the euphoric effects typically tend to be less intensive than those produced by opioid drugs and opium, more and more drug users still seek to use Kratom.

Digestive Damage & Liver Liabilities

85th thing you need to know...

The Journal of Medical Toxicology published a study stating Kratom use can lead to adverse side effects in the gastrointestinal tract (*i.e. upset stomach and vomiting*). It based its report on an individual who took Kratom for only 15 days without the presence of any other causative agents.

There have also been issues reported concerning liver injuries linked to Kratom ingestion. One report described the case of a young German who incurred impaired flows of bile within the liver after taking high doses of Kratom powder for just a couple of weeks.

Psychological Problems

86th thing you need to know...

The physical aftereffect symptoms of Kratom use can peak to their prominent states but they eventually fade away within a week. Its psychological side effects can be just as typical, but sometimes, they can be more detrimental.

These damaging effects may include addiction, aggressive behaviors, anxiety, crying, decreased libido, delusions, episodic panic, hallucinations, intensive mood swings, lethargy, paranoia, psychotic episodes, and suppressed appetite.

Waging Withdrawals

87th thing you need to know...

Some of the long-term users of Kratom may have difficulties giving up its regular use. They perceive a hard time to cope up with anorexia, bone and muscle aches, insomnia, jerky limb movements, psychosis and restlessness, which are the common withdrawal symptoms that follow upon a cessation of Kratom use. Nonetheless, while symptoms of Kratom withdrawal can be distracting and annoying, they do not exhibit debilitating pains as in the symptoms of opiate withdrawal.

88th thing you need to know...

Kratom withdrawal symptoms usually disappear after 1 to 3 days. Their common descriptions mostly connote to being short-lived and benign.

89th thing you need to know...

The upside for users amidst their Kratom dependence is that they continue to remain sound, fit, and trim. Besides having good health, they can still exercise normal functions, especially in their social interrelationships with others.

In fact, a Malaysian study showed no significant impairments in their performances of social functions and responsibilities.

Chapter 8: Legalities & Liabilities

90th thing you need to know...

Kratom is legal in most countries like the U.S.A. Although the U.S. Food and Drug Administration (FDA) has long released an importation alert cautioning the negative aftereffects of regular Kratom use in humans, the botanical wonder still enjoys unregulated status in most states in the U.S.

91st thing you need to know...

Kratom is only banned in six of the US states—Wisconsin, Vermont, Tennessee, Indiana, Arkansas, and Alabama. This prohibition largely stemmed from a citation of drug officials at the U.S. Drug Enforcement Administration (DEA) that considered and included Kratom in the list of "Drugs and Chemicals of Concern."

92nd thing you need to know...

On the contrary, Kratom is illegal in the whole of Australia, Bhutan, Denmark, Malaysia, Myanmar, and Thailand. In Europe, several EU-member states, like Sweden, Romania, Poland, Lithuania, and Finland, have regulated laws over the use of Kratom. Some of these states and countries even impose severe penalties for the possession or planting of Kratom.

93rd thing you need to know...

The current Kratom ban and control in Malaysia is under the Poisons Act of 1953. Those found guilty of distributing Kratom leaves or preparations illegally can be fined or be sentenced to jail for up to 4 years. The cultivation of Kratom is, however, not an offense in Malaysia.

94th thing you need to know...

In Thailand, officials reclassified the Kratom Act 2486 of 1943 to be under the Narcotic Act in 1979. This reclassification stipulated the illegal act of possession, planting, importing, and exporting of Kratom leaves. However, many Thai officials consider the reversal of the 75-year old ban on Kratom with respect to its valuable and unparalleled performances in weaning off opium addicts.

95th thing you need to know...

In Ireland, the government has just recently illegalized Kratom. At present, authorities categorized it as a Schedule-1 drug, which bestows Kratom with the same illegal status as heroin.

Similar to the US-DEA citation, most of the Irish politicians who passed this new law have never probably heard about Kratom or its potent alkaloids.

Laws can change; and, they do change all the time; so, please ensure that Kratom is legal in the area where you live prior to using it.

96th thing you need to know...

Like the DEA citation and the events leading up to the Kratom ban in Ireland, the status of Kratom continues to be uncertain.

Social Standing

97th thing you need to know...

The most important thing to consider before using Kratom is whether you are educated enough on the subject to make a responsible and well-informed decision.

98ᵗʰ thing you need to know...

In South East Asia, most users feel confronting rebuke from family and friends for 'engaging wastefully' in the habit of Kratom use. However, either certain acts of discrimination or stereotyping them as drug users never existed.

99ᵗʰ thing you need to know...

In the northern regions of Malaysia, users easily rely on and turn to use Kratom for its beneficial purposes due to its affordability and accessibility. In cases where users struggle against opiate withdrawal symptoms, they usually hinder themselves approaching and enrolling in government wellness facilities that may likely expose their identities. Instead, most of them enable self- treatments, which help them to avoid facing stigma, disgrace, or public disapproval of their drug dependency.

Therefore, fears of arrests by law enforcement authorities and censure from the community have pushed Kratom use to clandestine settings. Several reports in Thailand have highlighted a more recent and covert trend of a drug concoction used among its youthful generation— mostly, teenagers to people in their early 30s.

This latest drug concoction involves boiling Kratom leaves to serve as a primary base for a cocktail tagged as,"4 × 10." It is essentially a composition of Kratom tea, ice cubes, Coca-Cola, and cough syrup.

Kratom's Kismet: Future Fate

The practices of Kratom use in both the opposite sides of the world have moved gradually away from their traditional Western and Eastern applications—treating an array of physical maladies and enhancing physical endurance—towards newer uses with much potential promises.

100th *thing you need to know...*

One significant potential that the Kratom plant holds is its development as a viable treatment choice for opiate dependence. Recent findings insinuate its strong viability option by the huge volumes of Kratom purchases from online sources by at least 40 million Americans struggling from opiate withdrawal and suffering from chronic pain. Since 2013, the numbers keep growing steadily and there seem to be no signs of any letdowns in the near future.

101st thing you need to know...

People "in the know" view Kratom as an economical alternative therapy to more expensive, yet, less effective prescription treatments for the self-management of opioid withdrawal, as well as relieving pain. These claims only merit serious and further scientific research and investigation, particularly for the benefit of developing countries... and most of all, to the multitude lurking in ignorance.

Conclusion 2

Studies indicating Kratom's potential as a harm-reduction tool, most notably as a substitute for opioid addiction are still not enough to satisfy our question of whether Kratom is safe to use.

Both the scientific community and governments around the world truly need to perform extensive research and development studies about its uses and effects in order to form a precise and comprehensive understanding about Kratom. While the intriguing topic of completely banning or controlling Kratom keeps on heating up, some governments seem hell-bent to determine new laws while others simply remain hesitant to look back at the precautionary measures and side effects of taking this botanical wonder.

For some users, the negative mental health effects of Kratom—primarily withdrawal symptoms—appear to be relatively milder compared to those of opioids. For other indiscriminate users, withdrawal can be highly uncomfortable and it becomes more difficult to maintain abstinence.

Its pleasurable and euphoric effects only give rise

to its addictive qualities. The addiction is usually associated to a developing tolerance, especially for heavy or daily users. Actually, almost none of the plant's essential components are addictive. Therefore, in reality, the chances of Kratom abuse are very low.

However, among many users, Kratom enhances the mood and relieves anxieties, stress, and depression. Several users also rely on Kratom for its effective pain-relieving qualities and inhibiting properties of suppressing symptoms of various anti-inflammatory diseases.

These actual user results should urge, on one hand, medical researchers and mental health or substance use clinicians to consider resuming further investigations on the negative side effects of Kratom to humans, and for good reason! On the other hand, policy makers and regulators must conduct a sweeping review of current laws and regulations of Kratom use before arriving to faulty conclusions and decisions.

The positive effects on the health and lives of many users are as significant to consider. It can truly be life preserving for opiate abusers to use Kratom in a positive manner and along a regulated short-term duration to end fatal drug dependencies.

In ending, the key point I would like to reemphasize is to be diligent and responsible enough to do your own part. Investigate and perform your own research. Consider all factors involved, including your mental and physical conditions. Seek consultations with your physician as well prior to using Kratom.

Never hitch on the bandwagon of media and promotional hypes. Only choose reliable and trustworthy suppliers. Know how they manufacture or process and source their Kratoms.

Cheap prices can be tempting, but quality must remain paramount.

Lastly, I hope you have enjoyed reading this book bundle and I would appreciate all your reviews.

www.ingramcontent.com/pod-product-compliance
Lightning Source LLC
Chambersburg PA
CBHW071544220526
45469CB00003B/915